Jump Into Nudism

Lucas Riviera

PLEASE NOTE

This book contains photos of nude people in everyday situations. This is not a pornographic book in any way, but it is filled with nudity. All images within this book comply with all United States Laws.

If you would like to get the version without pictures, send me an email request.

RIVIERALUCAS@GMAIL.COM

Thank you for taking this time to read about nudism. Hopefully this book will help get you ready to take the plunge into a better way of life.

I hope you enjoy this book.

-Lucas Riviera

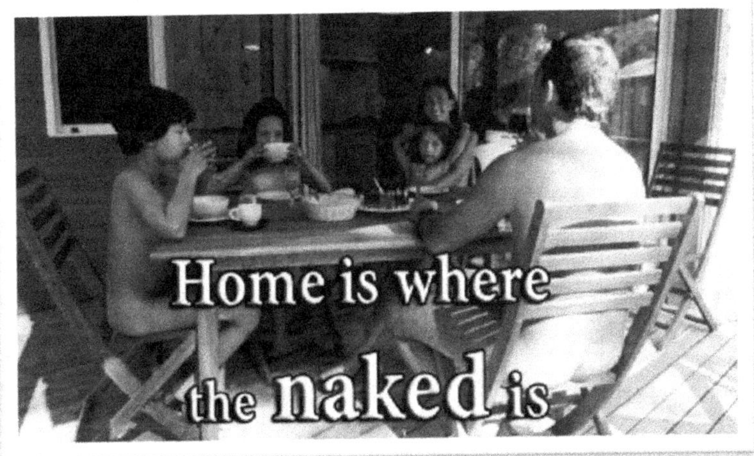

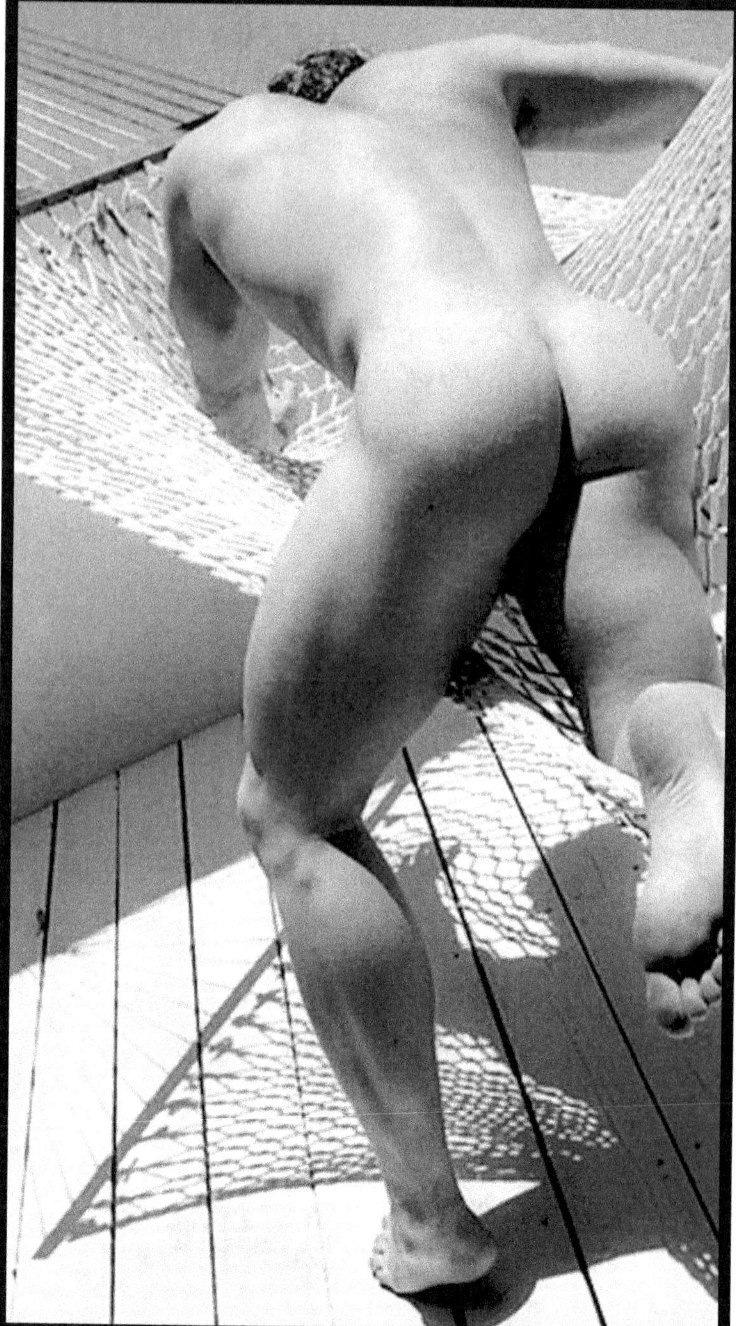

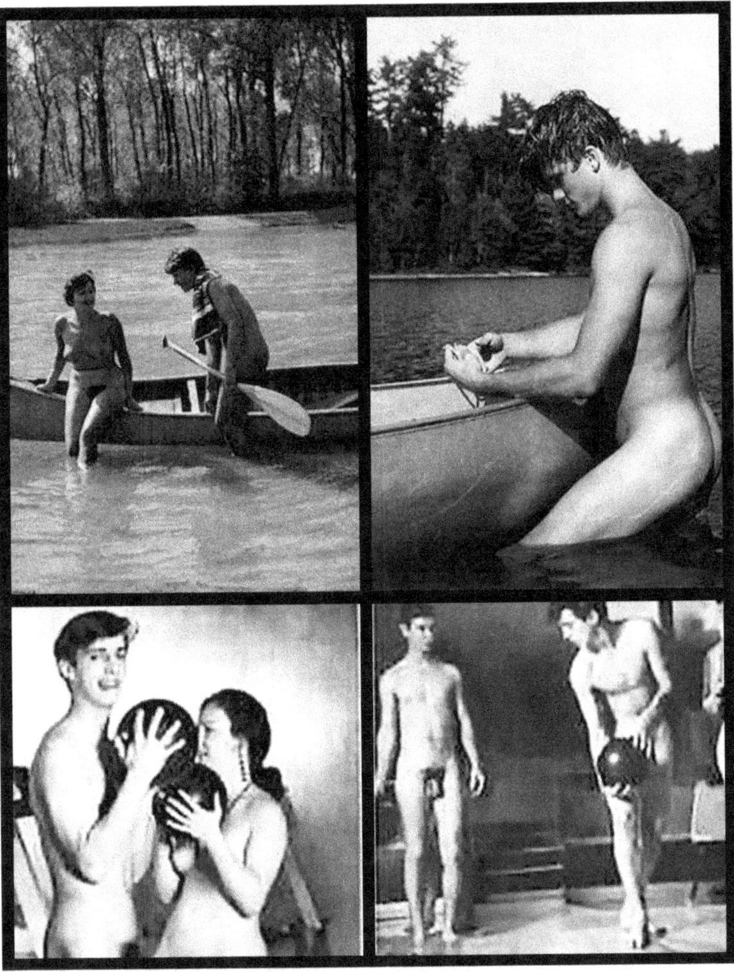

The History of Nudism

Nudity in social contexts had been practiced in various forms by many cultures throughout human history. In modern day societies, especially here in the United States, the most frequent type of social nudism comes in the context of bathing, swimming and saunas, but is typically gender segregated. However, in other societies around the world, and throughout history, nudism is normal at sporting events and competitions.

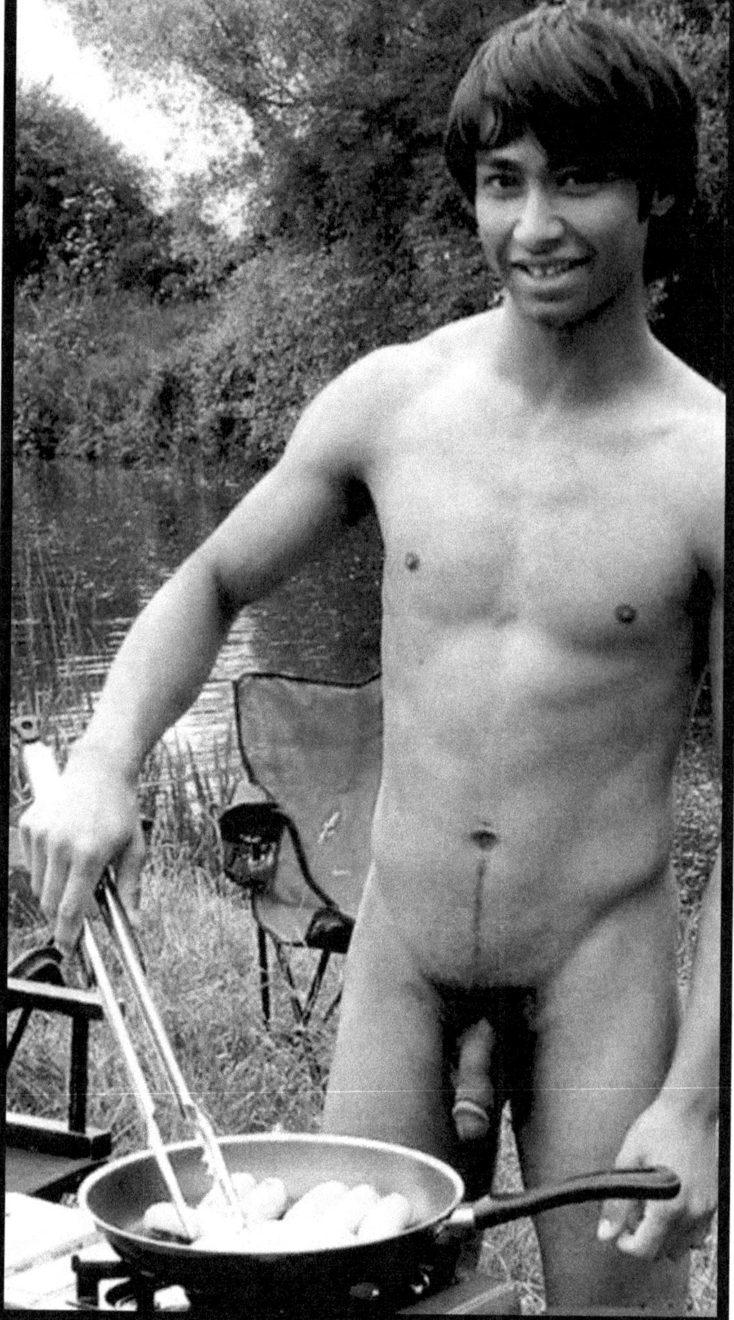

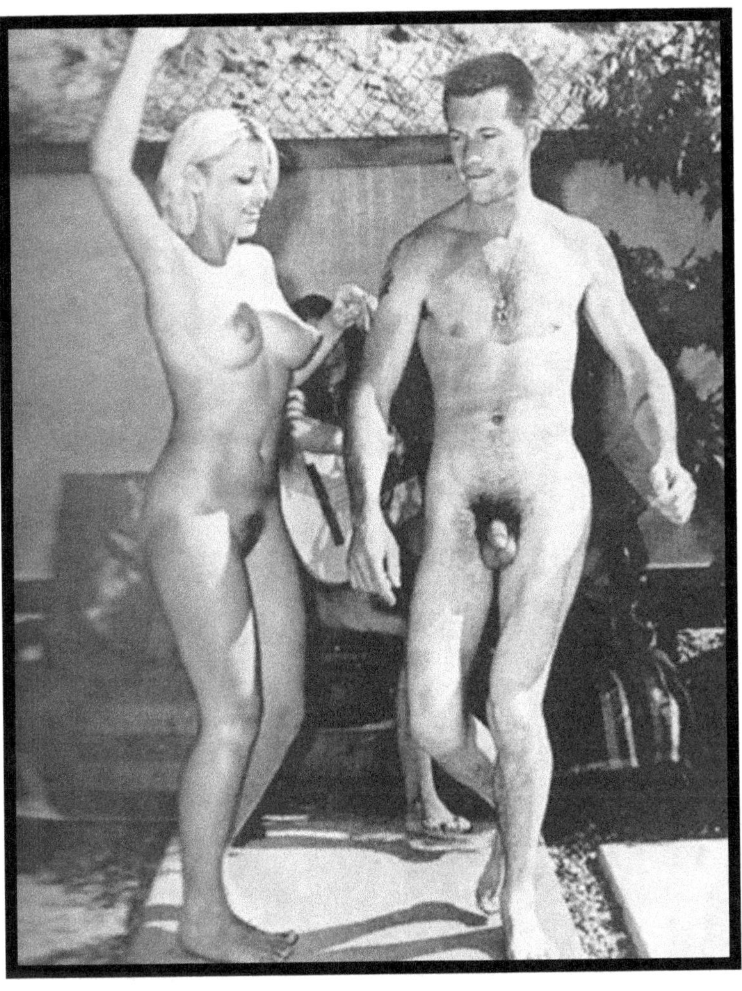

As far as my research has uncovered, the oldest record of a
nudist club, as we know them today, was established in India in
1891 by the British colonists. "The Fellowship of the Naked
Trust," was founded by Charles Crawford, and consisted of only
three members. However, the commune fell apart after the
British Government transferred him out of India.

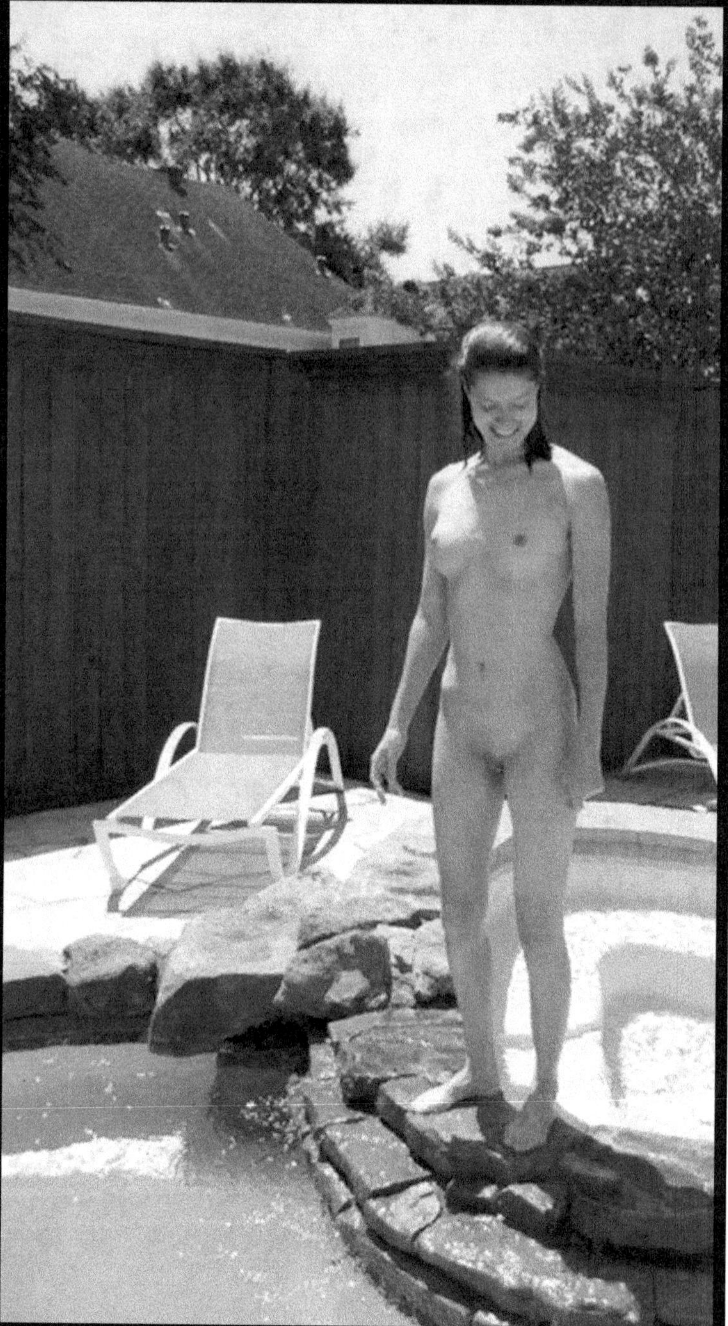

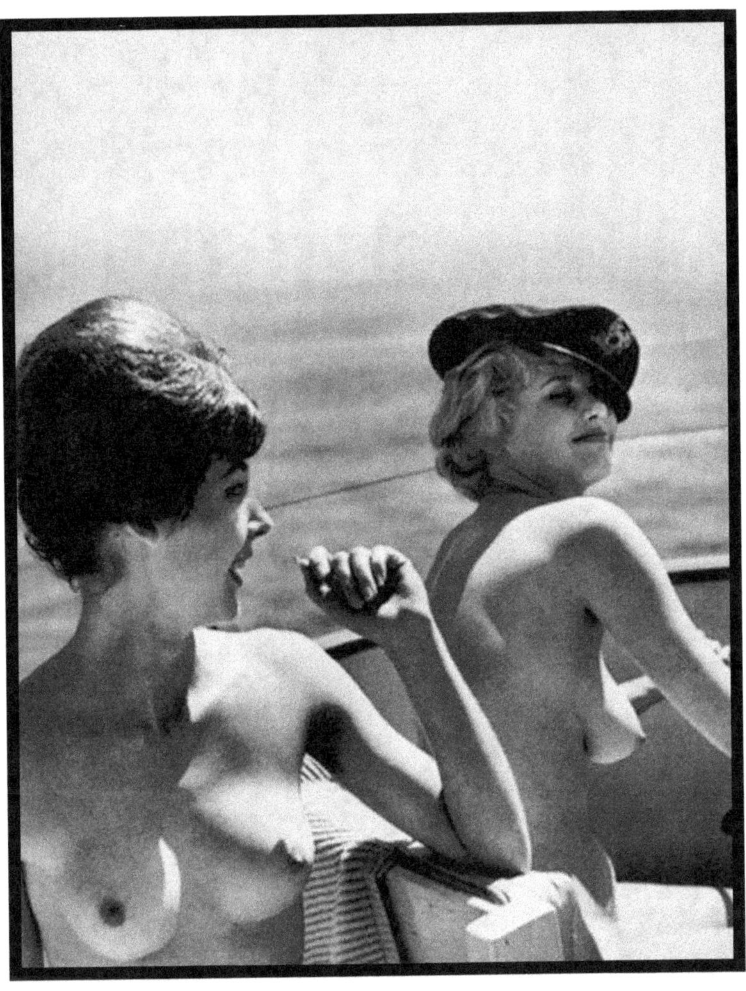

In the early 20th century, two brothers, French Physicians by the name of Gaston and Andre Durville, studied the effects of psychology, nutrition and environmental on the health of individuals, caused by nudism. Their studies convinced them in the benefits of natural foods and the natural environment; they then named this concept Naturisme.

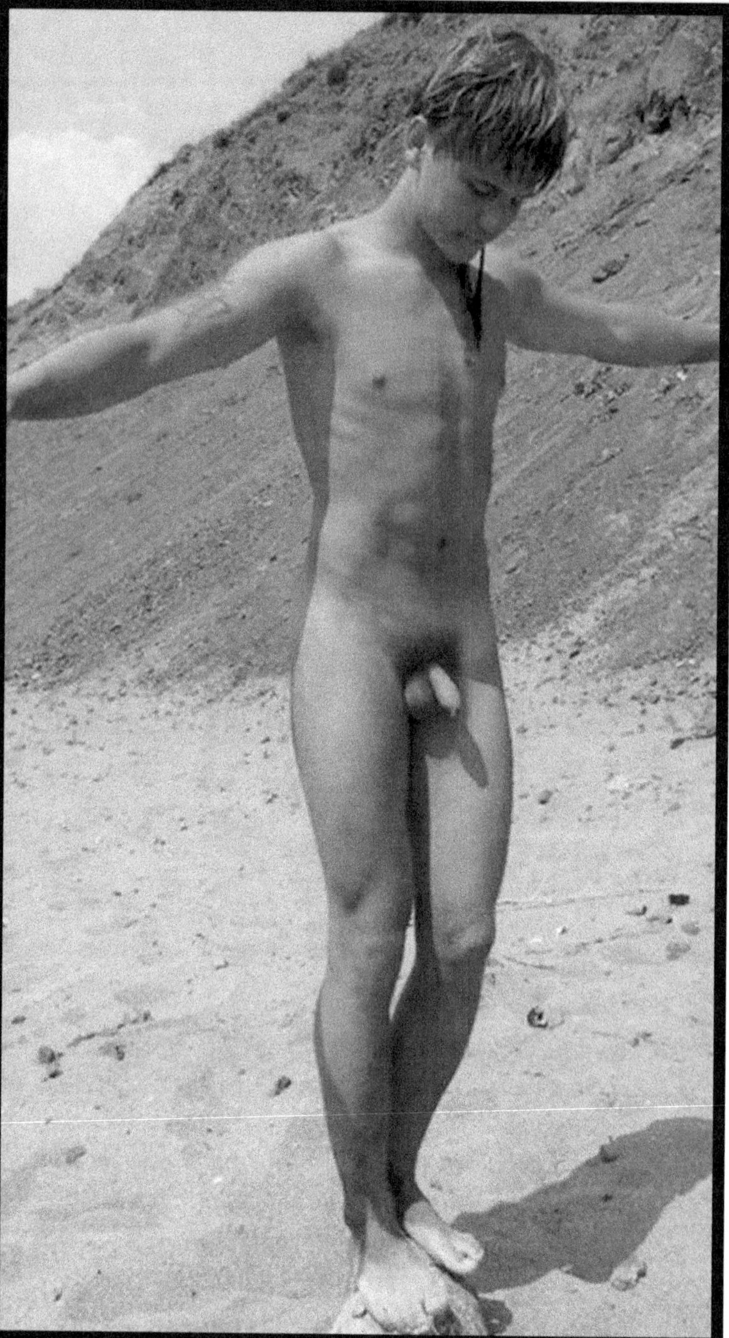

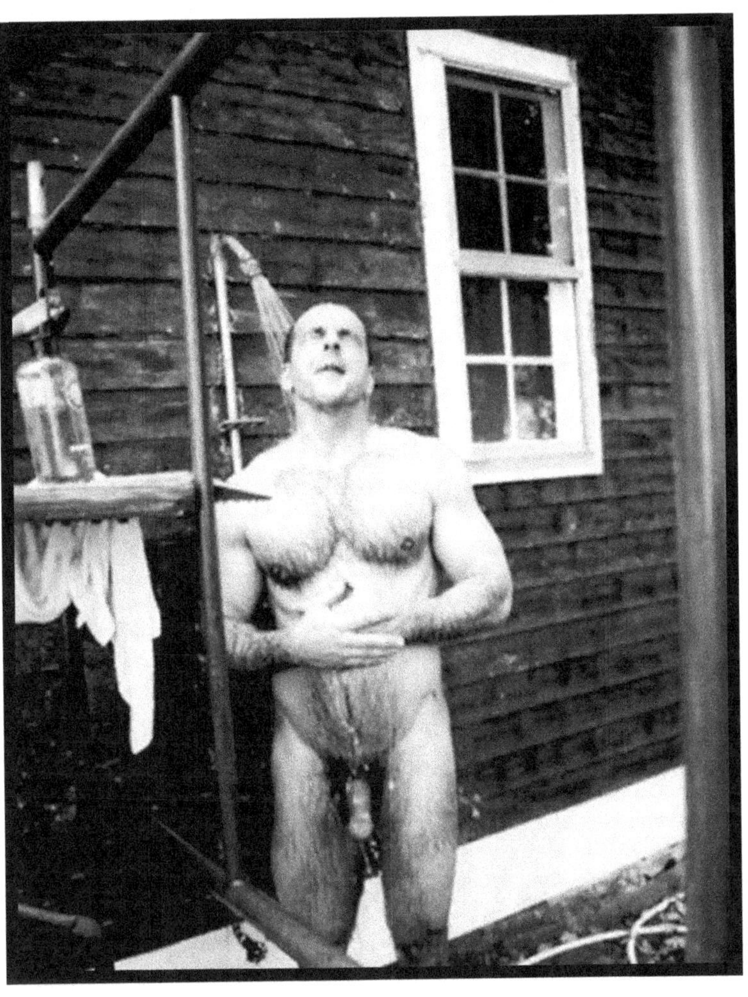

Nudism became more mainstream in the 1920's, as it spread through Germany, France and the UK. This was then brought to the United States, via German immigrants, in the 1930's.

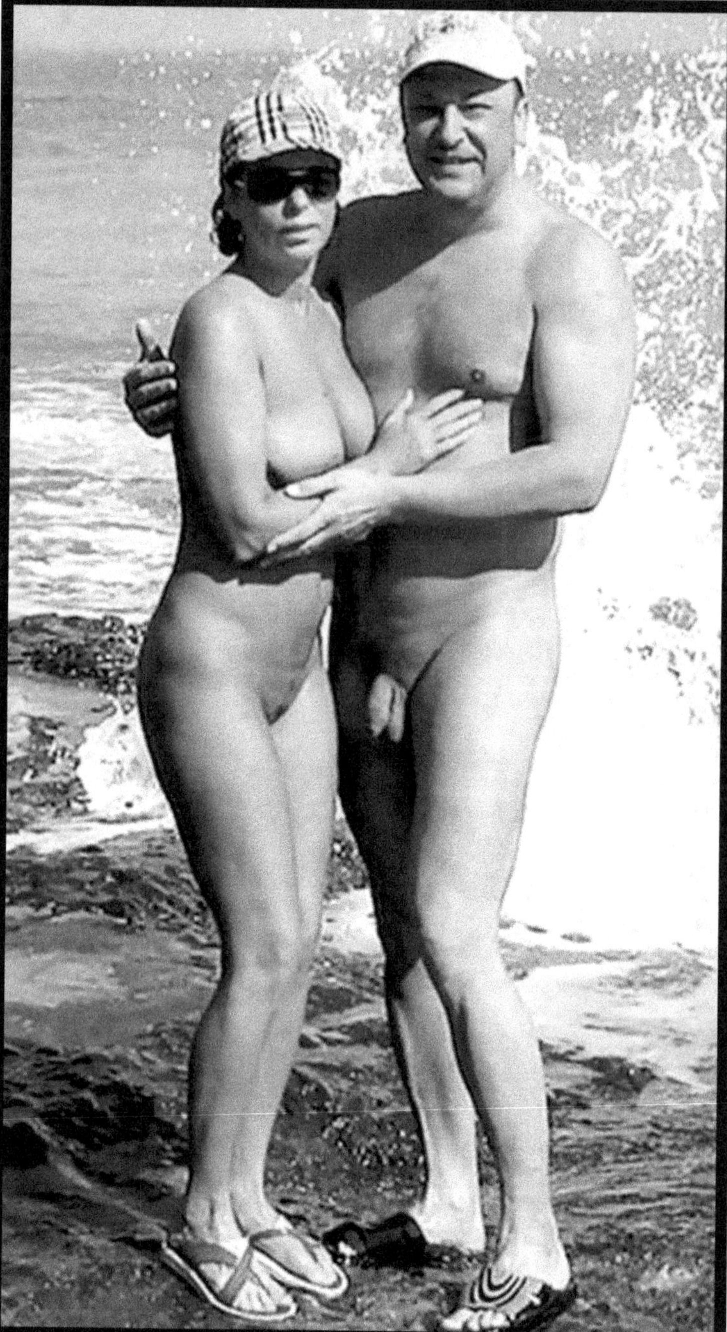

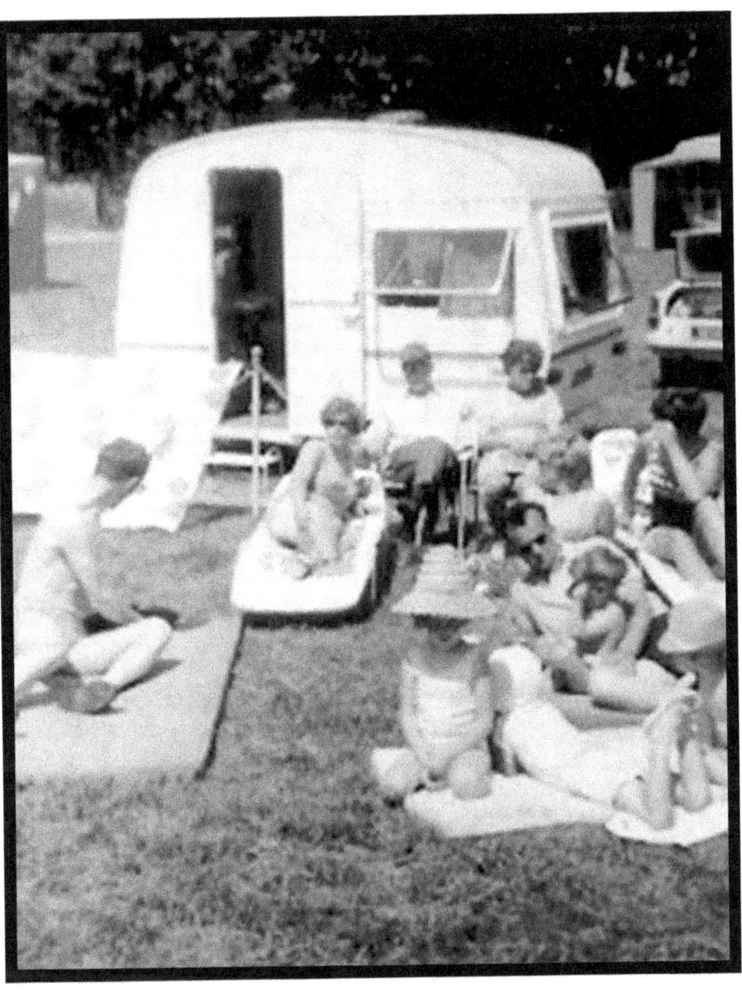

In 1951, nudism around the world was so profound that the communities came together to form the International Naturist Federation. However, many individuals preferred not to join a club, and in the years following 1945, there was a lot of public pressure to open specially designated, Nude Beaches.

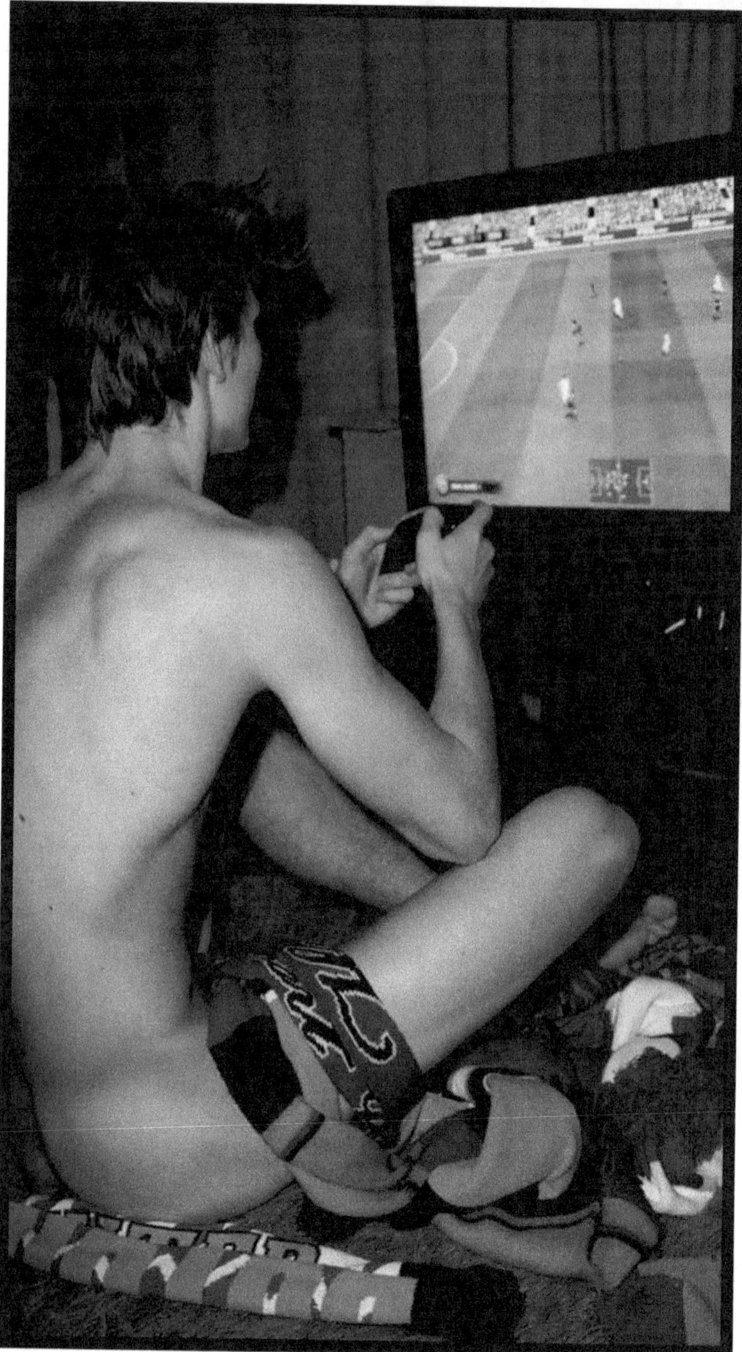

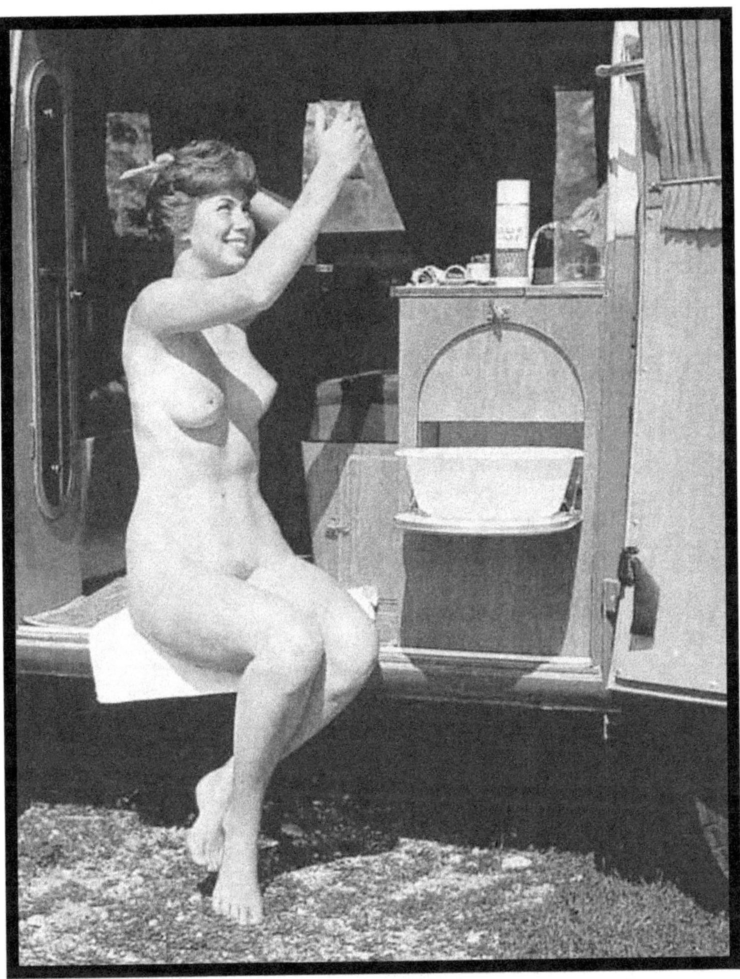

Common Nudism Misconceptions

The biggest thing that I hear is that people associate nudism with sex. In fact, in my experience, it is quite the opposite. Actually the biggest issue with the nudist community, in my opinion, is their prudish attitude towards sexuality.

For example, if a breeze was to catch a man in a certain way and he was to get a random erection, he can be asked to leave a resort or nudist beach.

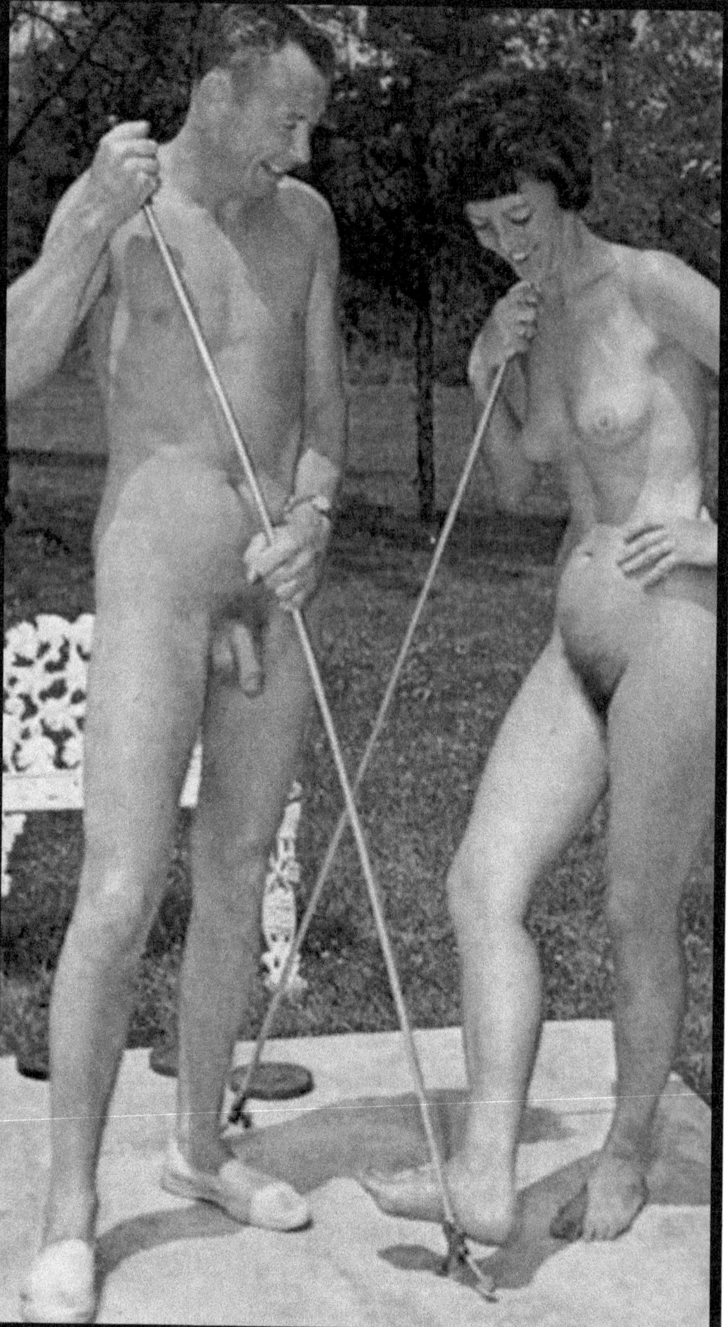

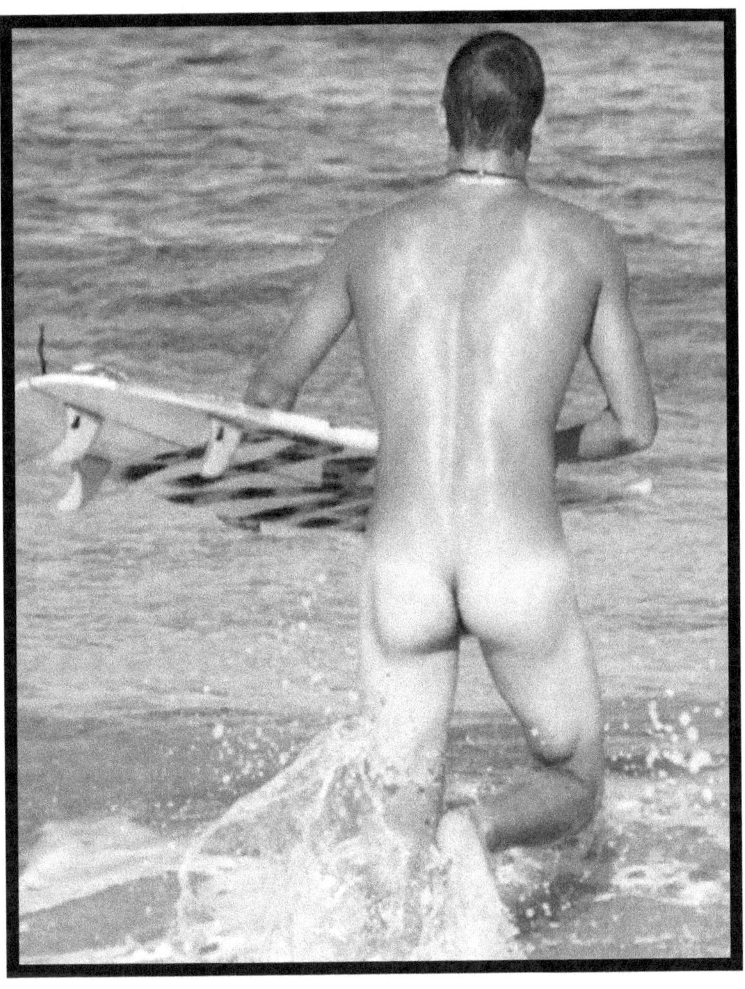

That brings me to misconception number two. Although I have never had this happen to me, I understand the fear, and before someone freaks out about that fear, the simplest thing on a beach is to just roll over in the sand until it goes away.

In my experience, someone who is really interested in nudism for its values, and not for the naked people, does not generally have this problem.

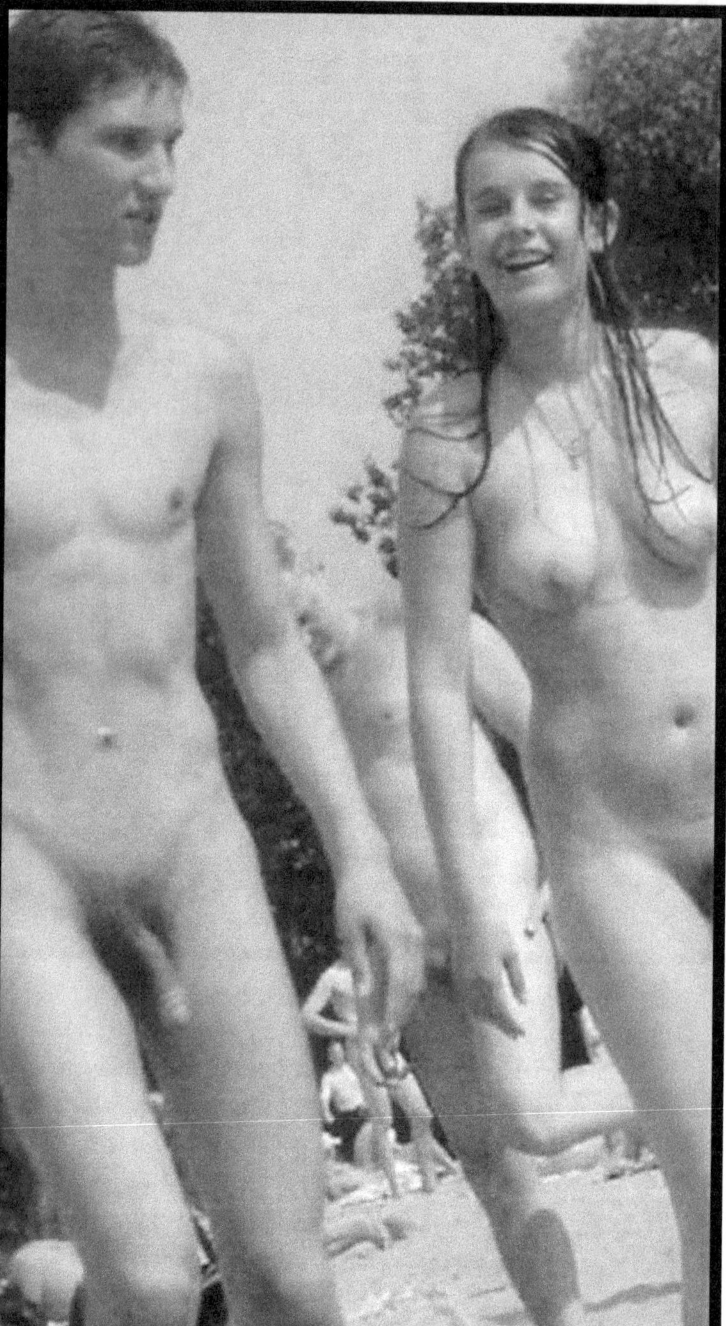

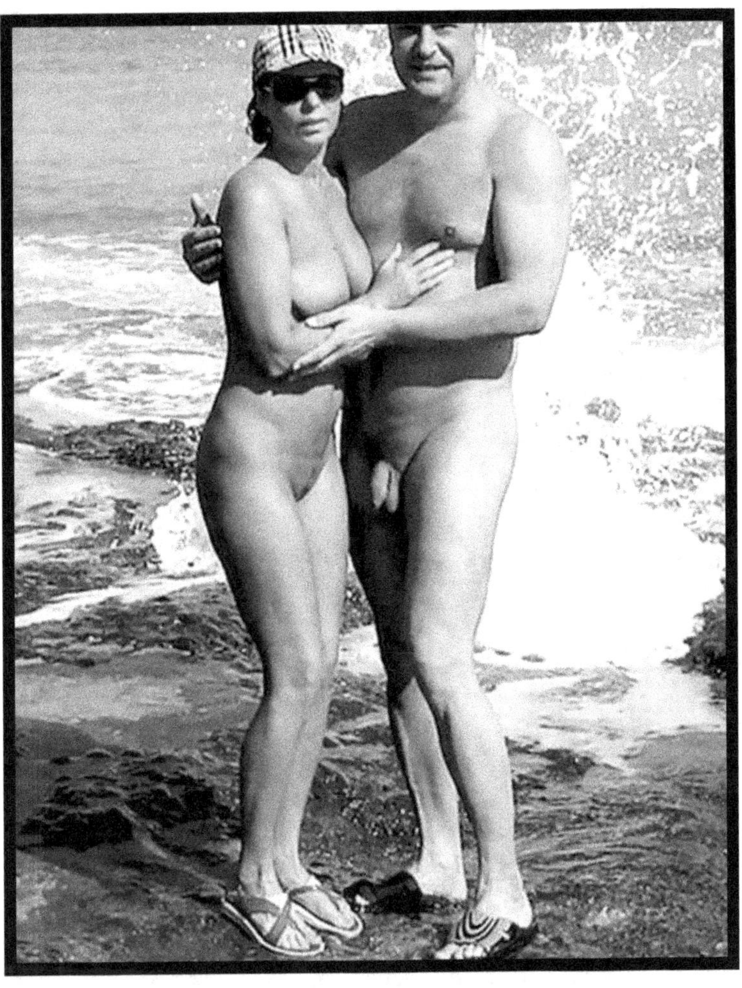

I have a friend of mine, who I was speaking to about nudism, commented that she didn't think she could do it; she always has to have on shoes, because she couldn't stand to walk around barefoot. I understand, and I agree, I always wear socks or shoes.

Let us remember that nudism isn't simply about being naked all the time, it's a lifestyle about being as comfortable as you possibly can.

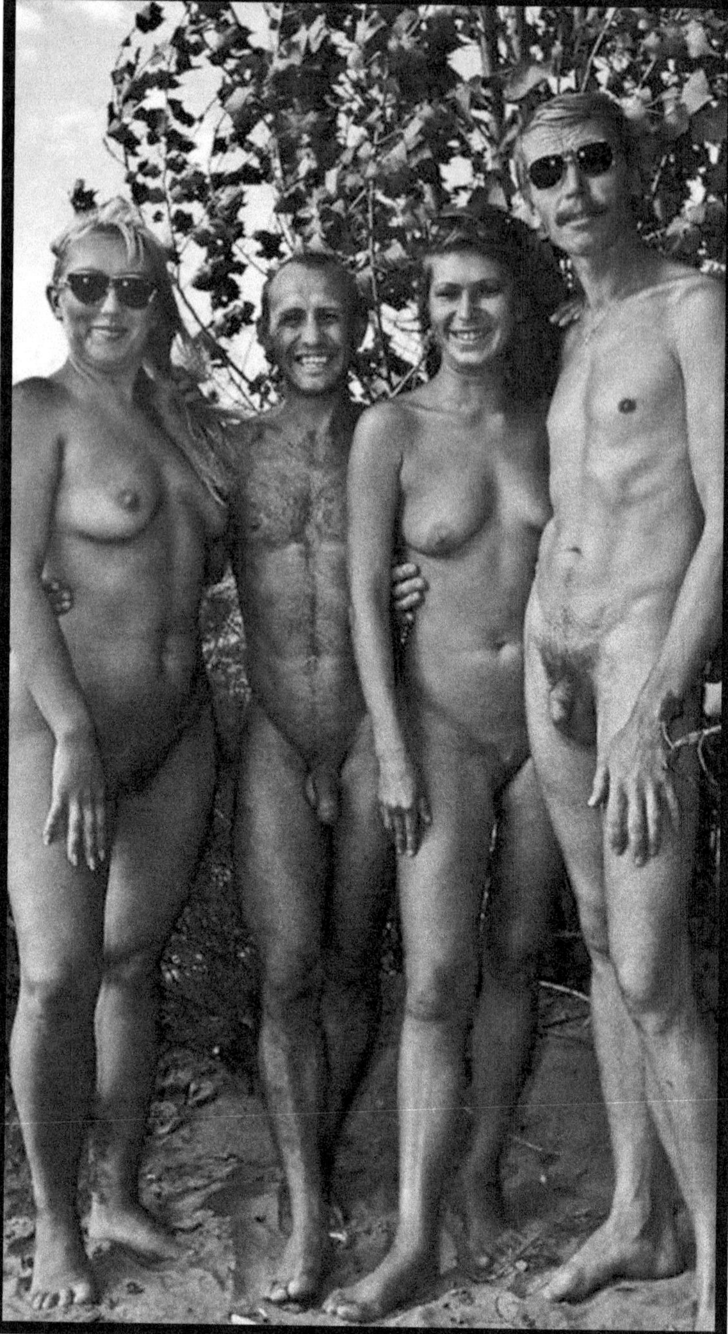

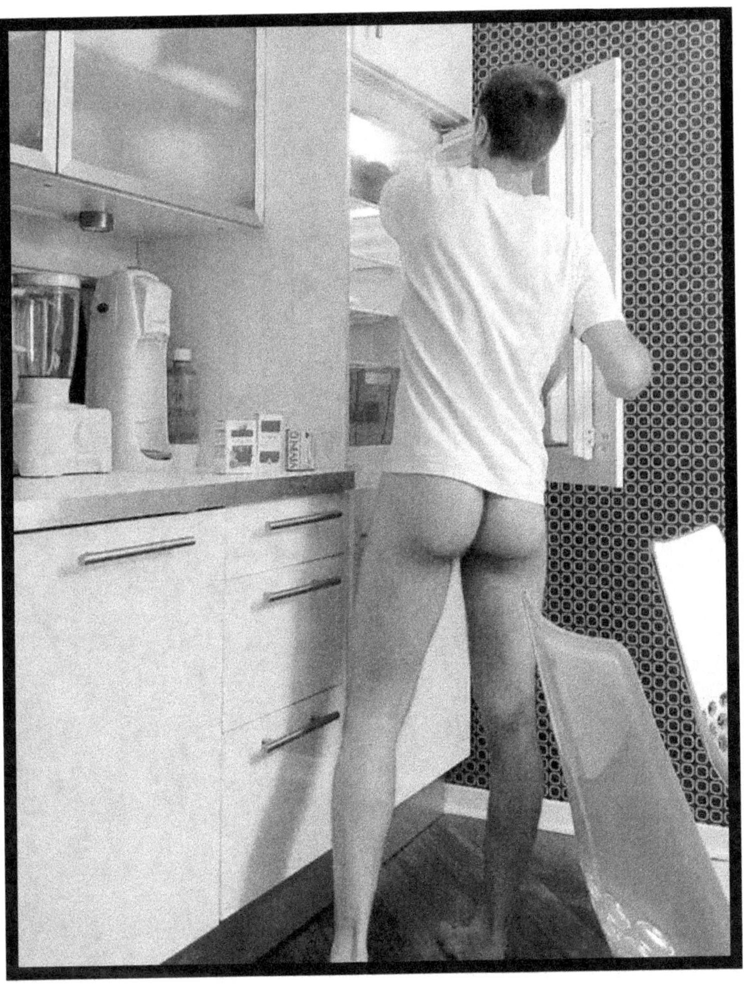

You do not need to be nude all the time to consider yourself a nudist. Nudism is a desire to be nude, or mostly nude. Let's be honest, unless you live on a nudist commune there is no way for you to be 100% nude all the time.

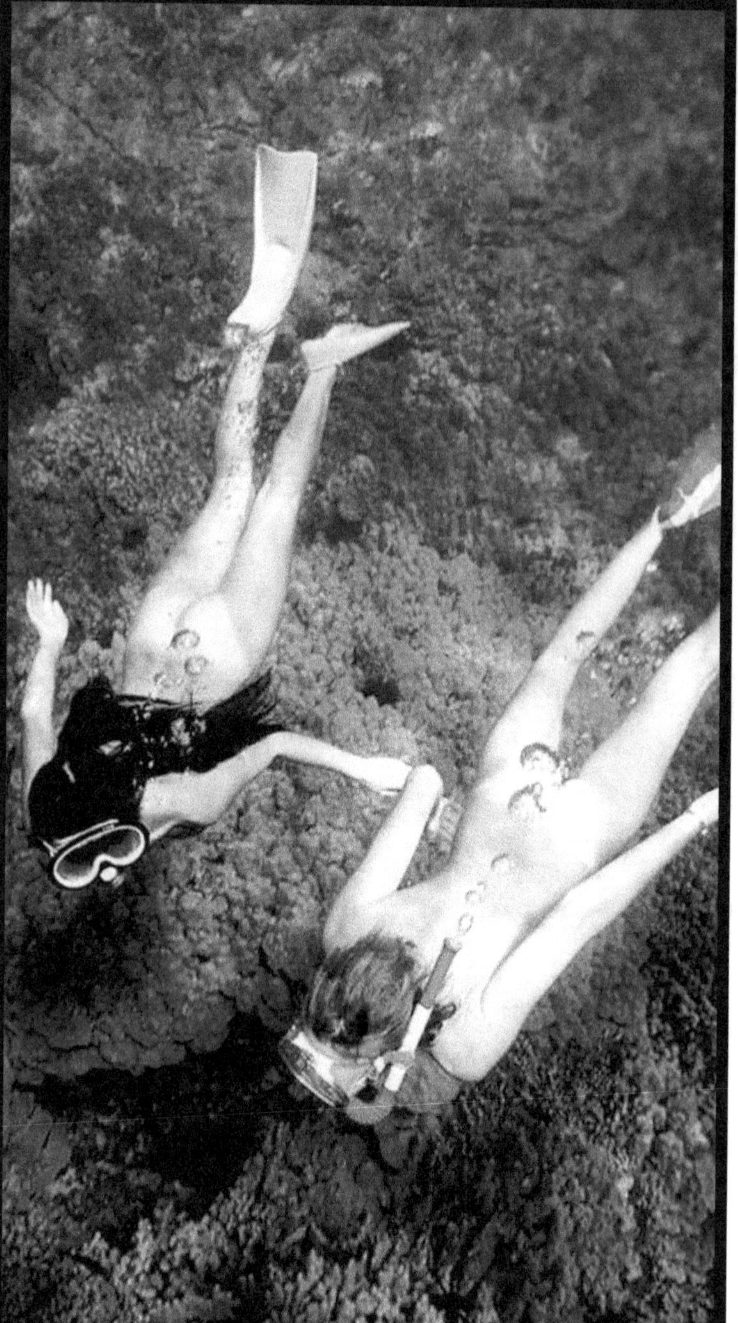

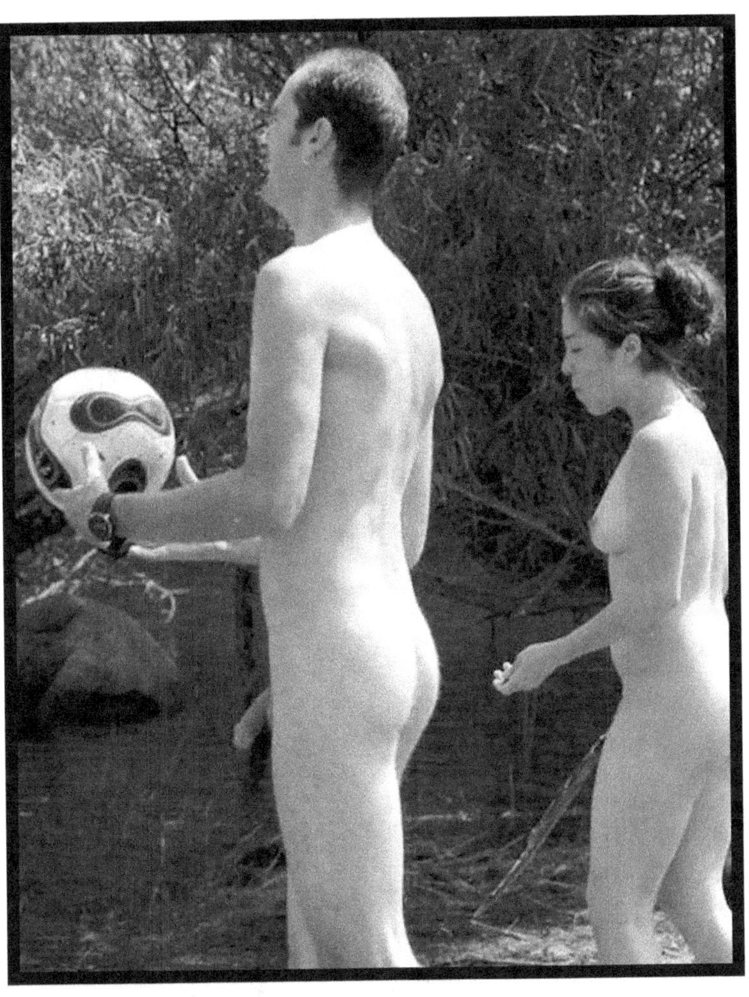

It is not a requirement to go to a nudist colony or nudist resort to consider yourself a nudist. Just like you don't need to play in a soccer league to consider yourself a soccer player, you don't need to belong to a nudist club or organization to consider yourself a nudist.

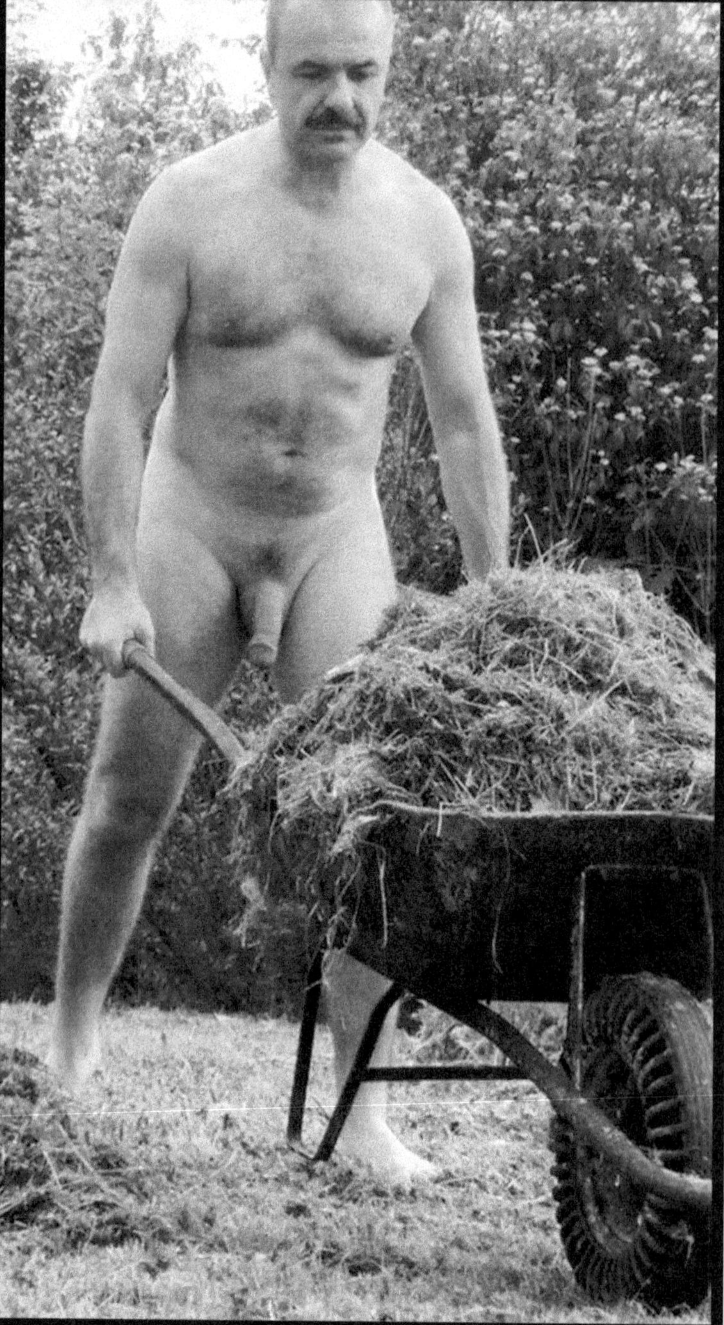

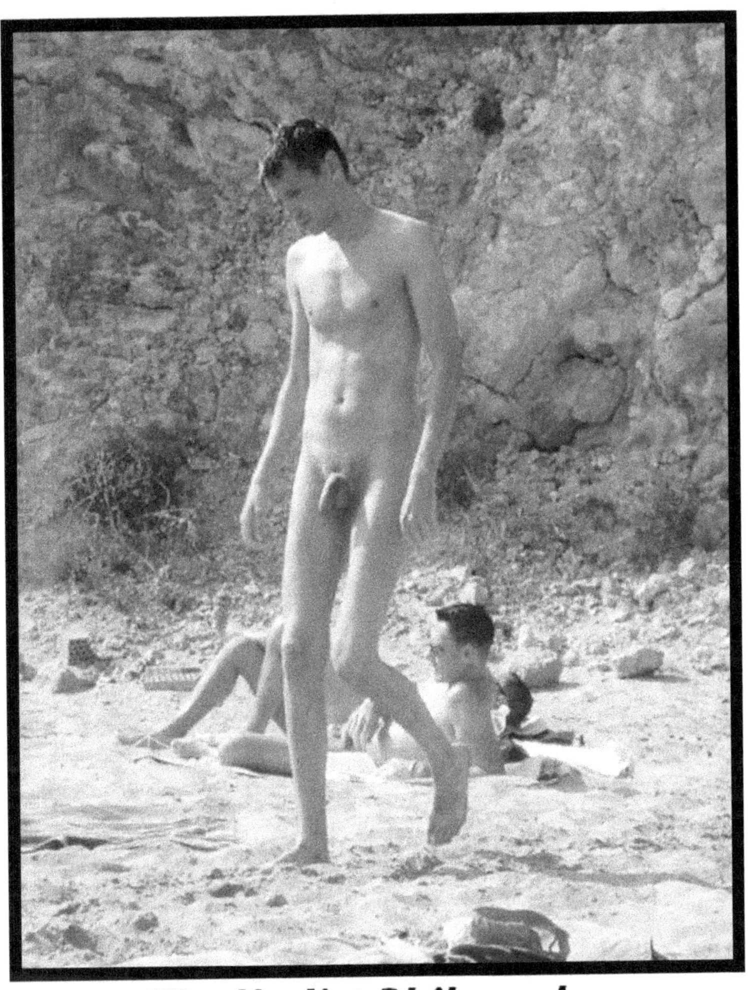

The Nudist Philosophy

Individuals have been forming nudist groups for a variety of reasons and purposes. In general, there is an understanding amongst Nudists and Nudist Organizations, that eroticism and blatant sexual acts have no place in nudism and are in fact directly opposed to its ideals.

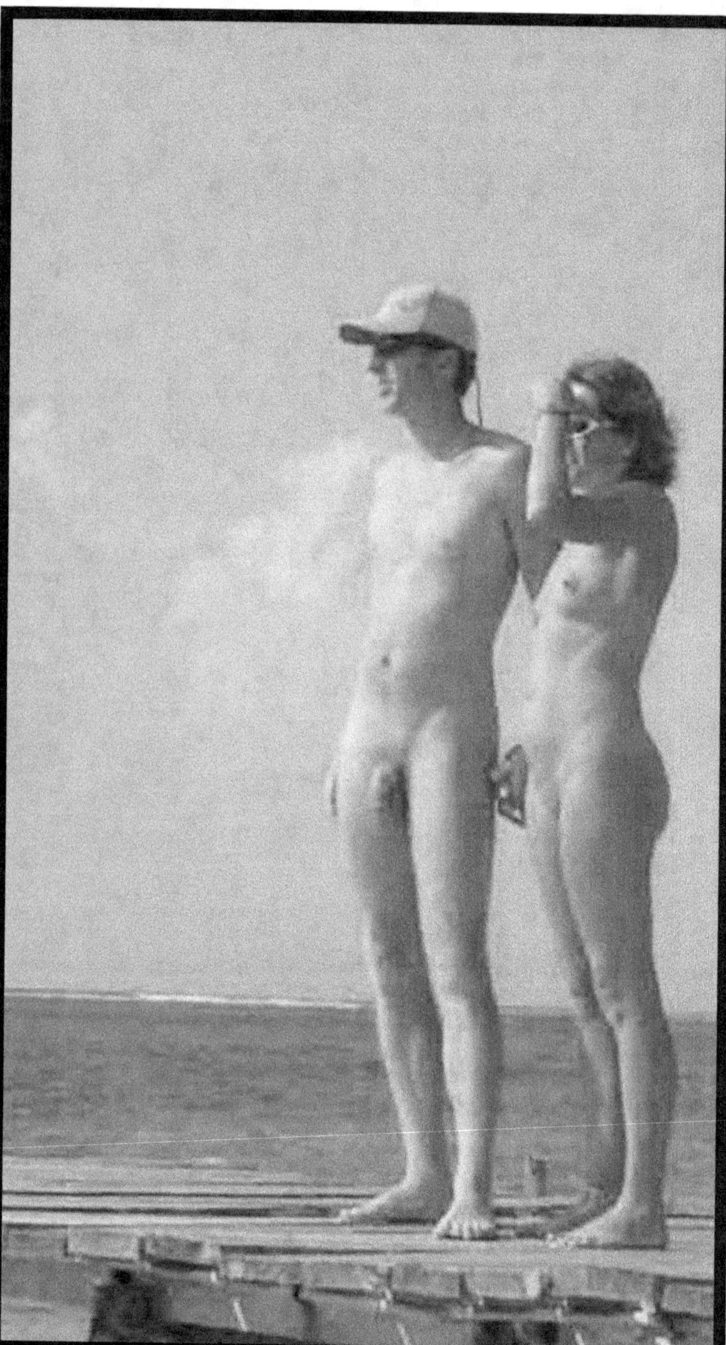

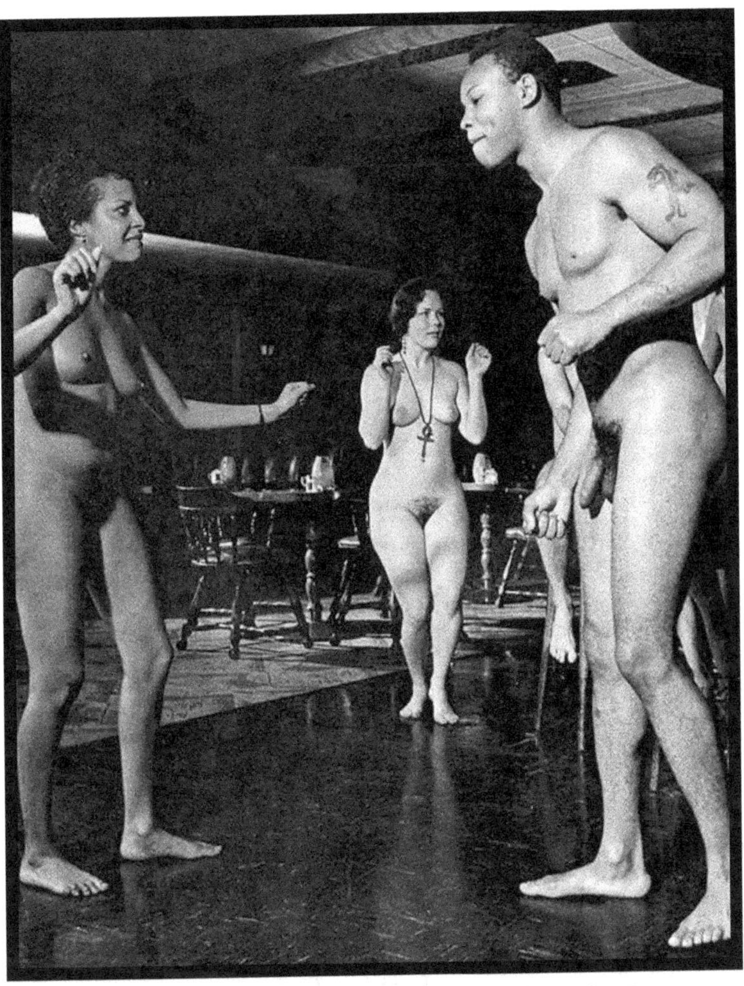

Some common arguements for participating in Nudism include:

• Heath – Bathing in the sun, fresh air and water.
• Psychological – being naked in groups makes all feel more accepted, and increases self-esteem.
• Spirituality – nudity, wellbeing, and direct contact to nature helps one feel closer to the creator.
• Equality – clothes build barriers, and social nudity leads to acceptance, regardless of differences in age, body shape, and health

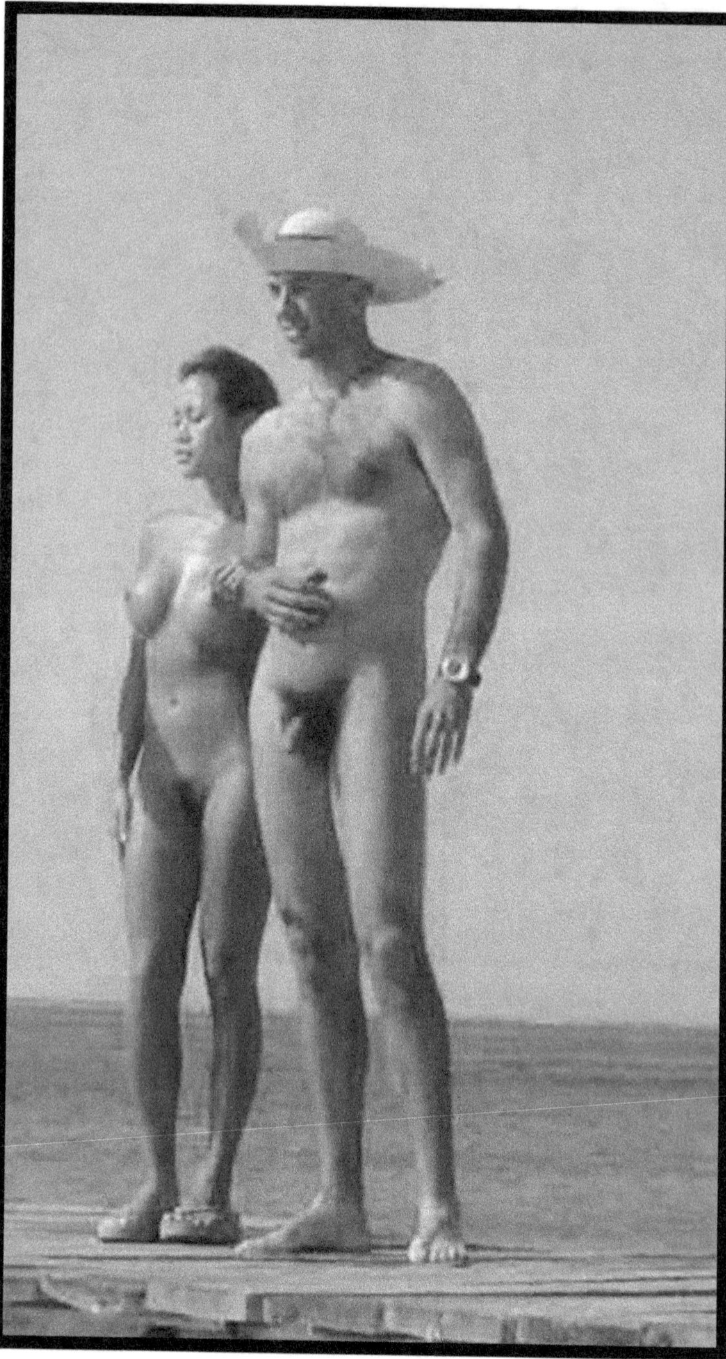

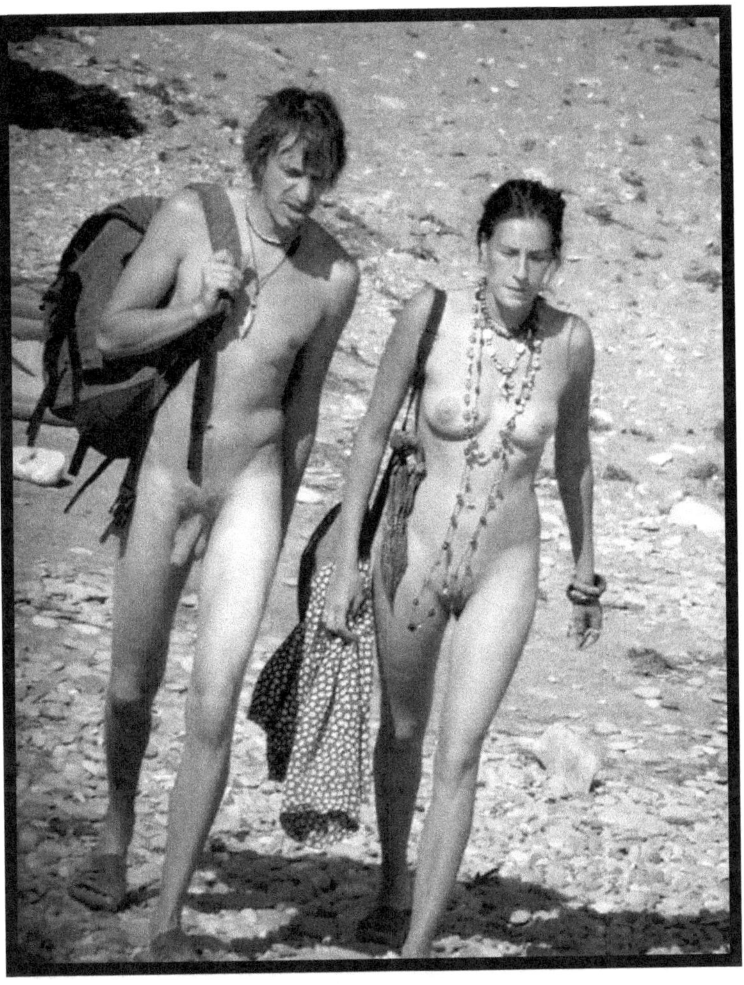

The great American writer, Walt Whitman, wrote the following pertaining to nudism, "Never before did I get so close to Nature; never before did she come so close to me... Nature was naked, and I was also... Sweet, sane, still, Nakedness in Nature!... Is not nakedness indecent? No, not inherently. It is your thought, your sophistication, your fear, your respectability that is indecent. There come moods when these clothes of ours are not only too irksome to wear, but are themselves indecent."

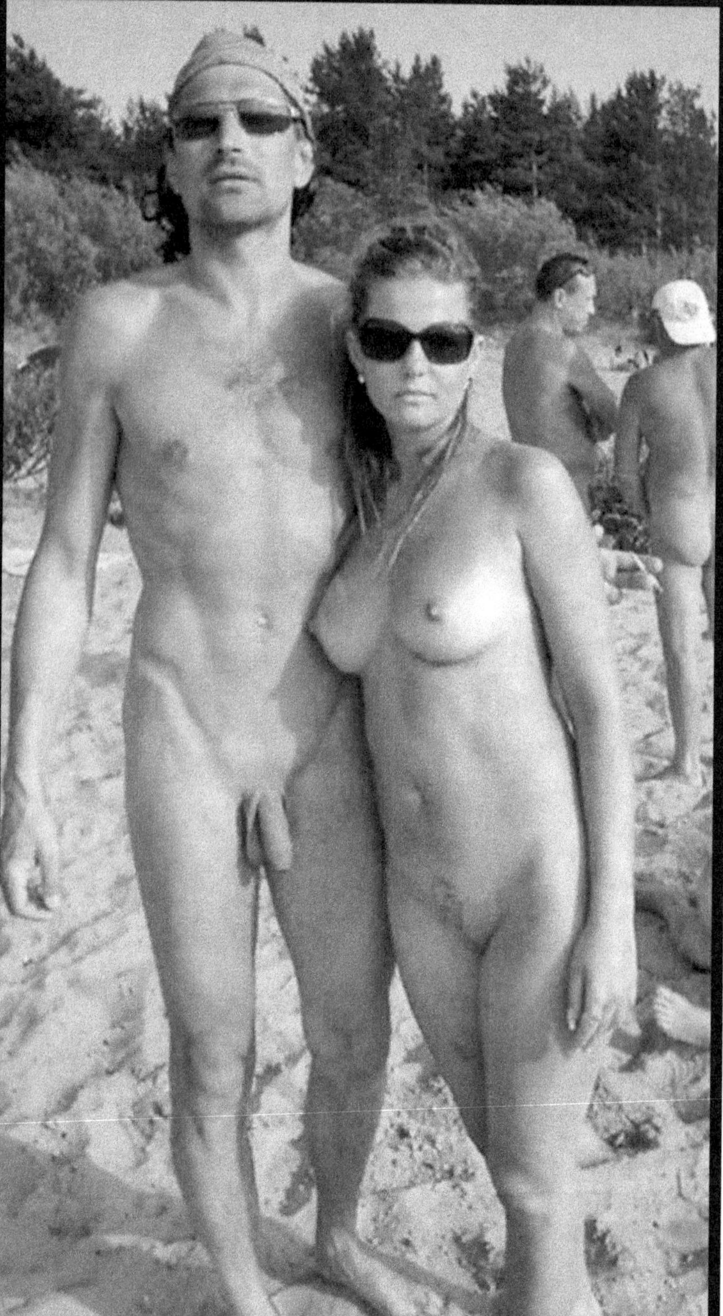

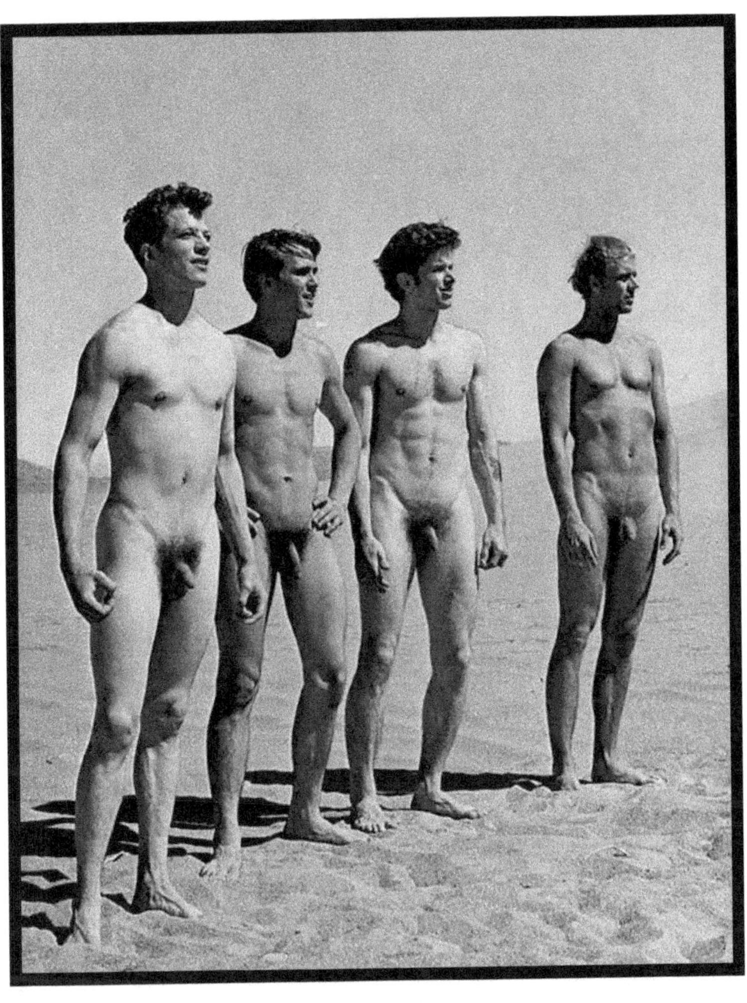

Henry Thoreau also wrote, "We cannot adequately appreciate this aspect of nature if we approach it with any taint of human presence. It will elude us if we allow artifacts like clothing to intervene between ourselves and this other. To apprehend it, we cannot be naked enough."

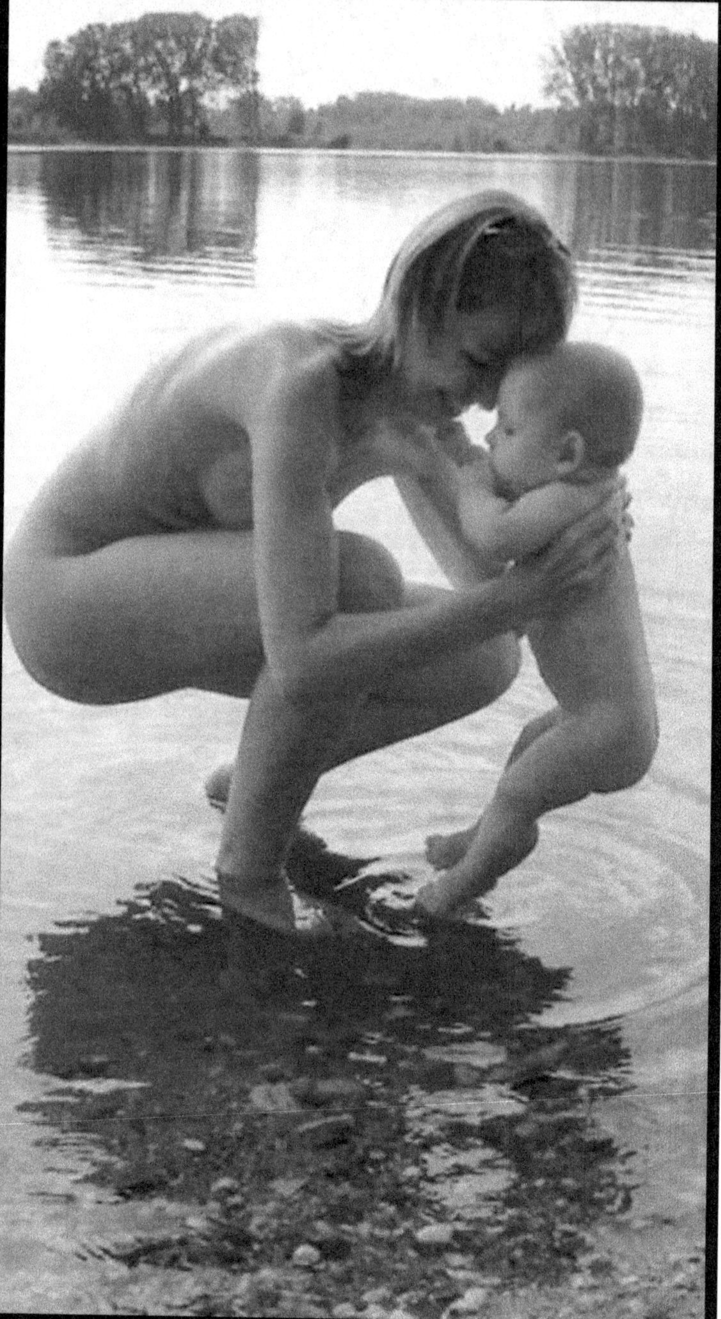

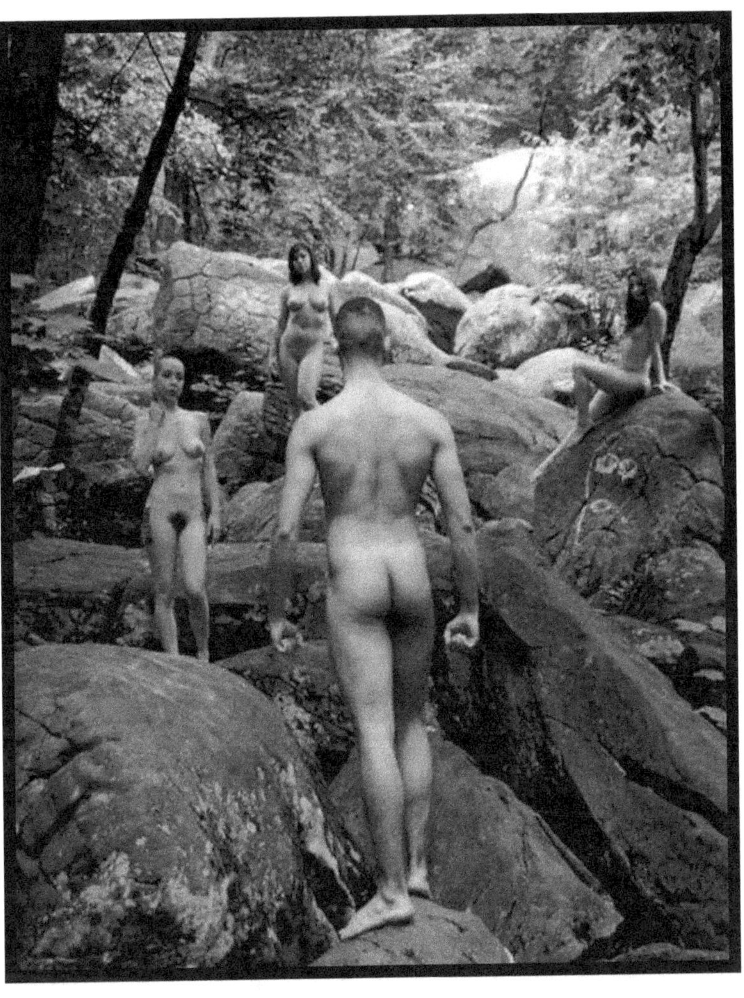

Nudism went through a big movement via literature in the late 1800s, which also influenced are if the era, especially the works of Henri Matisse, a French painter, who was known for his use of color and works as a draughtsman.

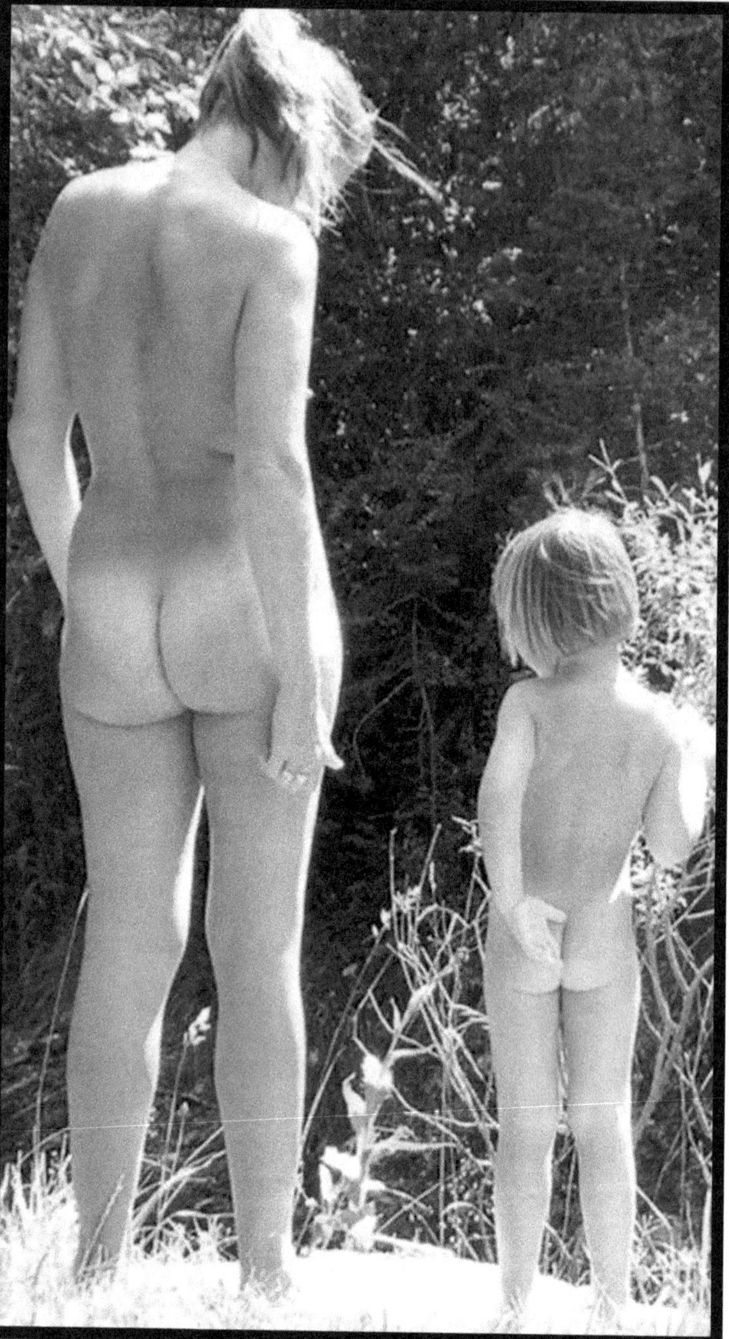

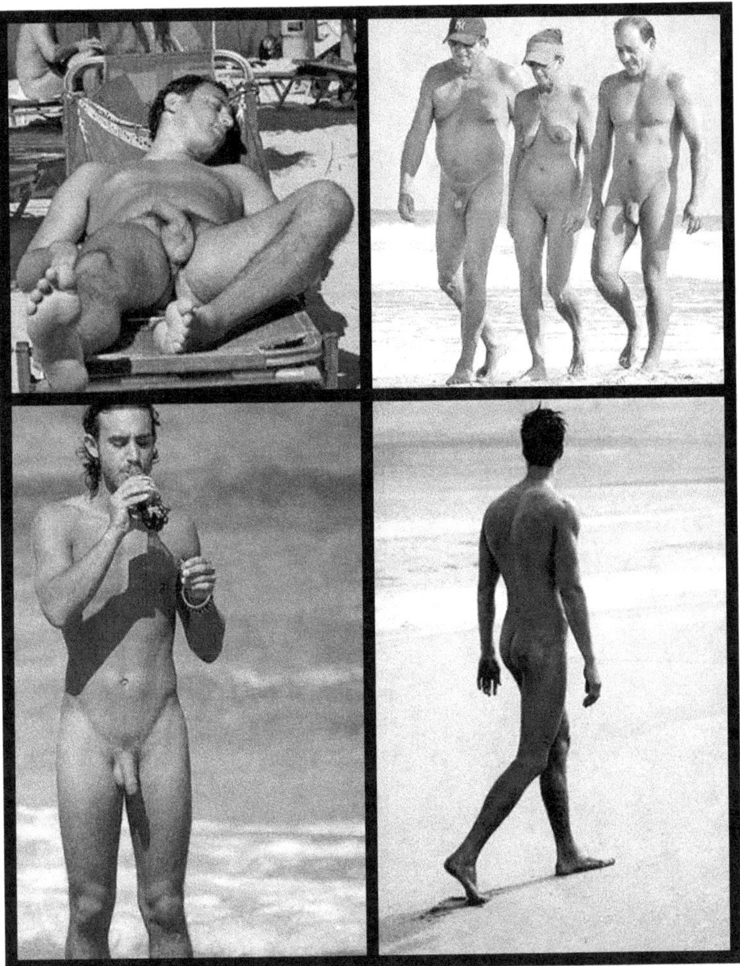

Health Benefits of Nudism

Sunlight has been shown to be beneficial to one's health, as sunlight enables the body to develop Vitamin D. Recent medical studies have shown that the skin's exposure to sunlight also prompt the body to produce Nitric Oxide, which helps support the cardiovascular system and also produce serotonin.

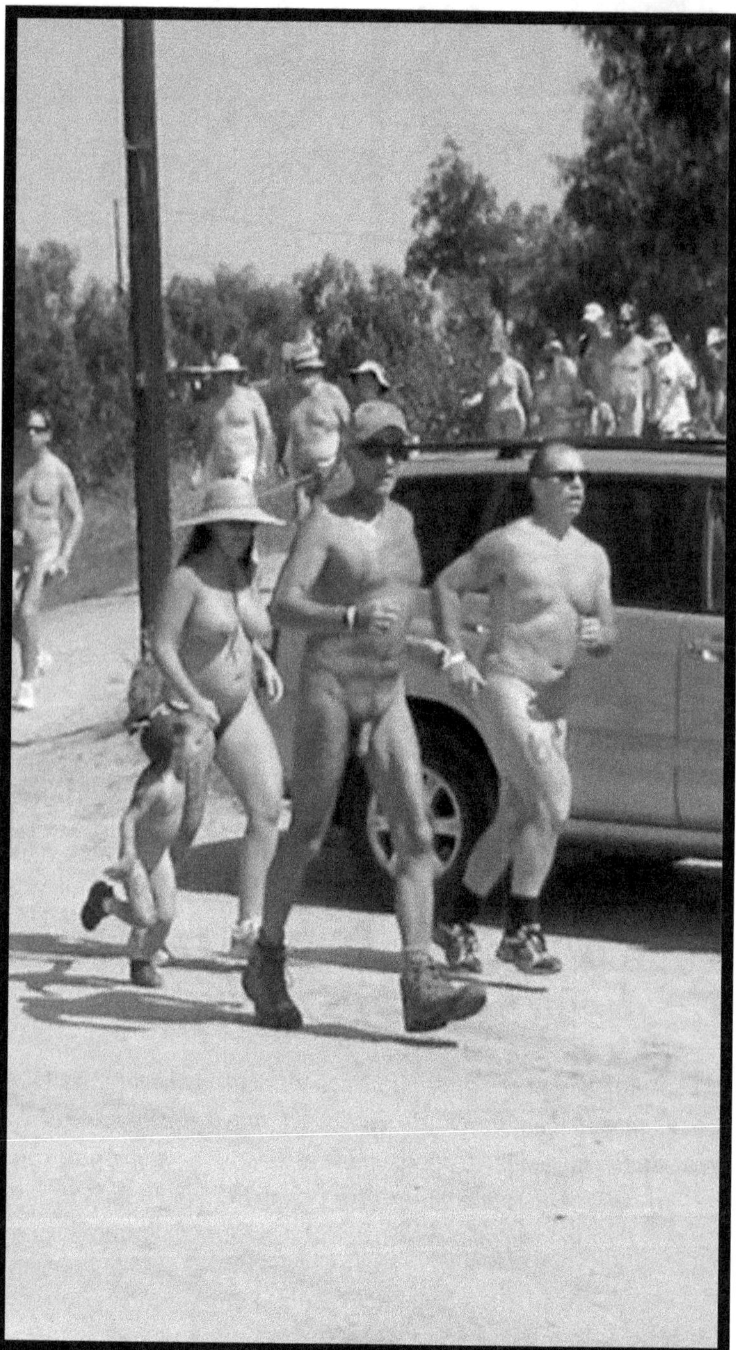

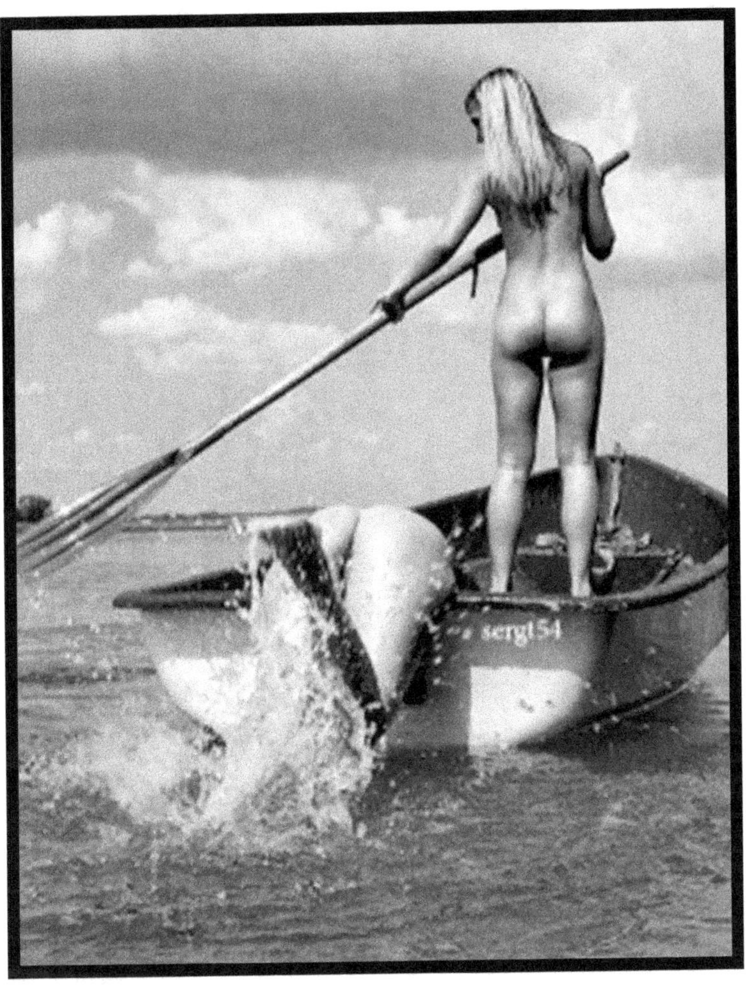

While it is well known that the Sun can be harmful to the body in large doses, the harsh effects can be tempered by products such as suntan lotion and other methods to reduce the harmful effects, but maximize the positive ones.

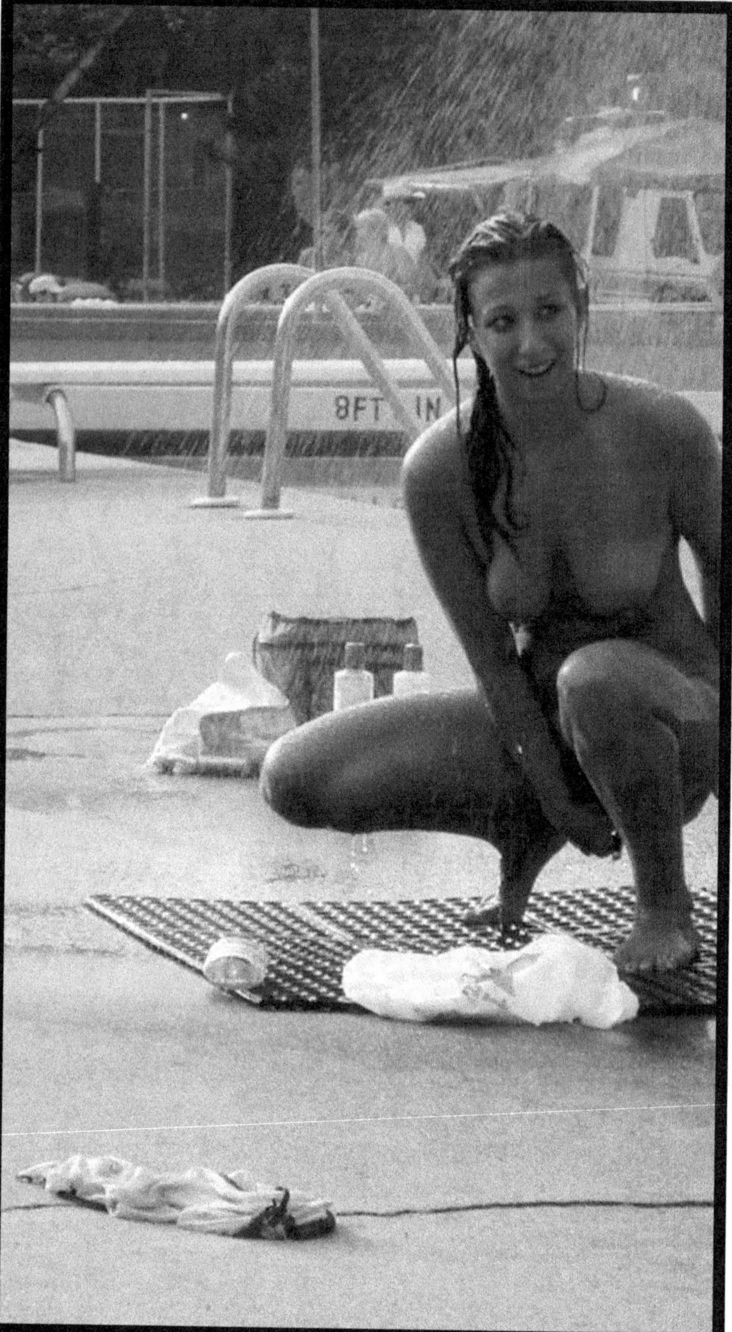
8FT IN

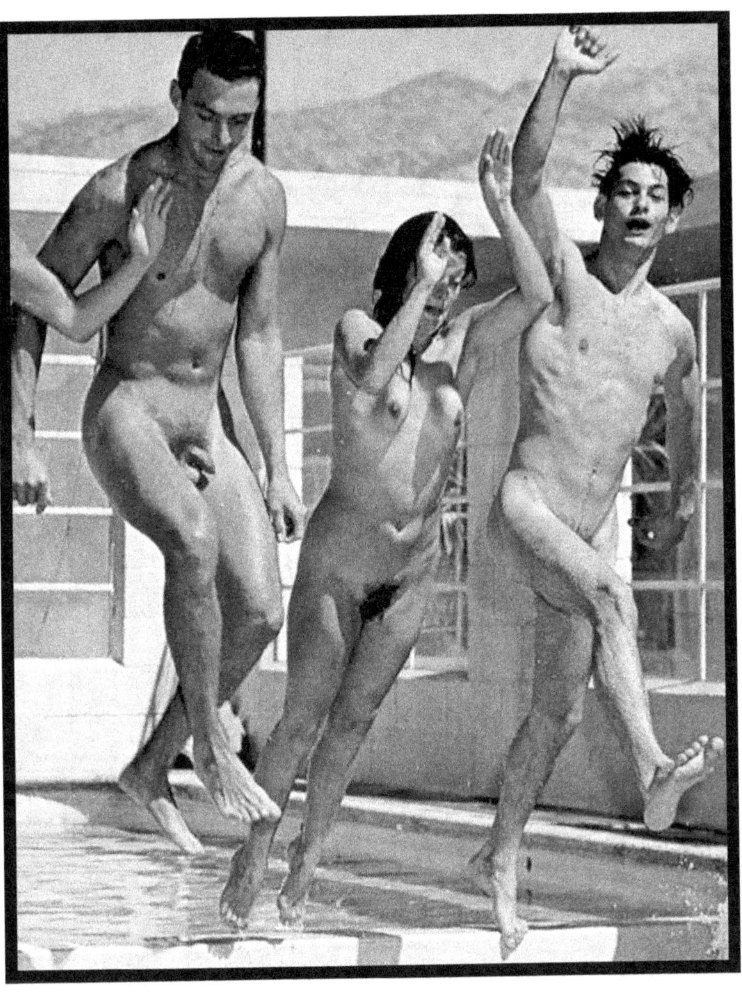

There are also documented psychological benefits of nudist activities, including a more positive image, higher self-esteem and a generally happier life.

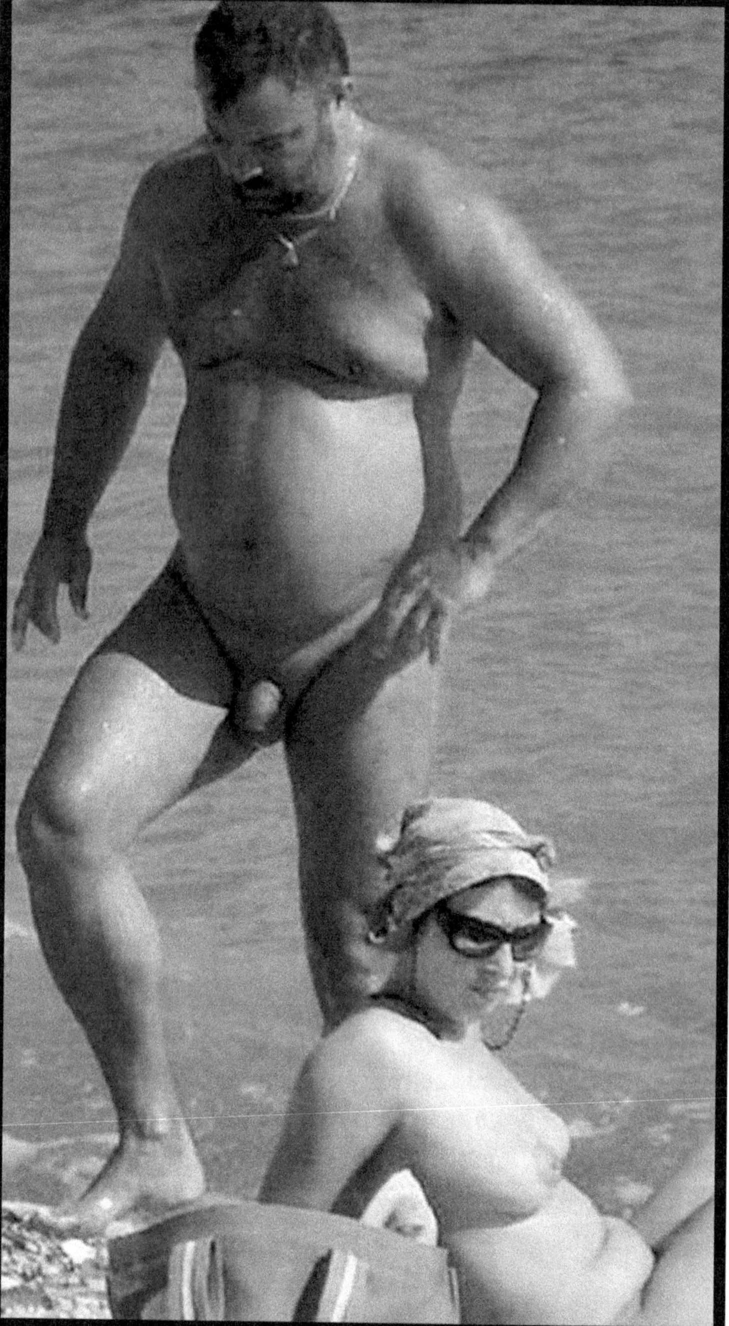

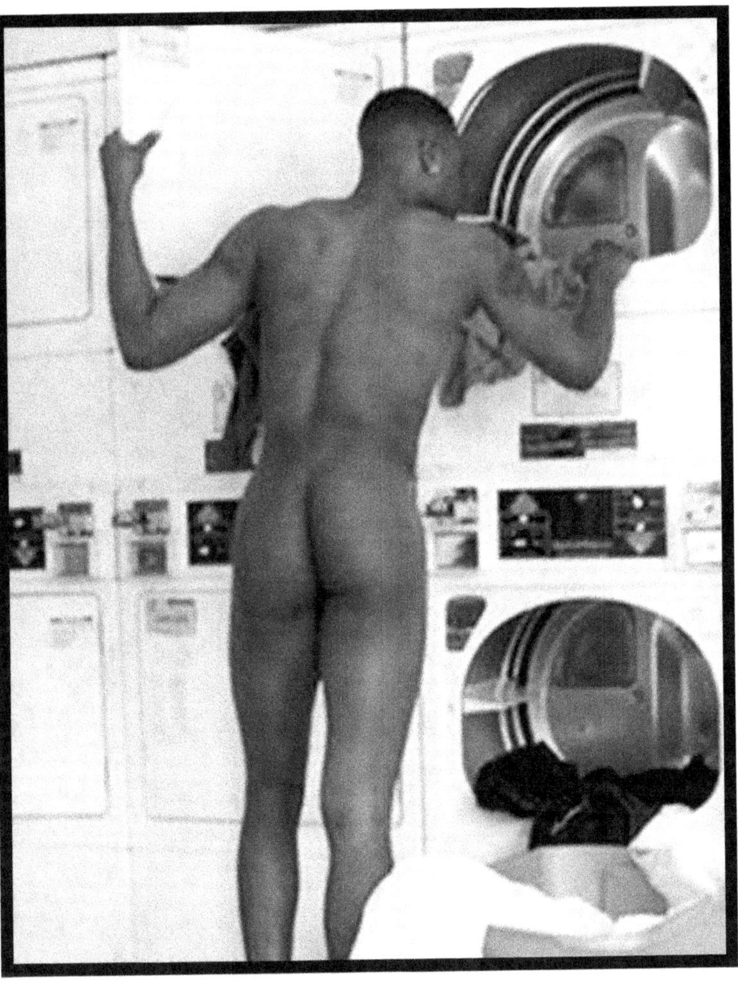

One of the things that my research never brought up, but that I noticed on my own, is that when I don't wear clothes, I don't have to do laundry. This in turn, saves me money and helps cut down on water usage.

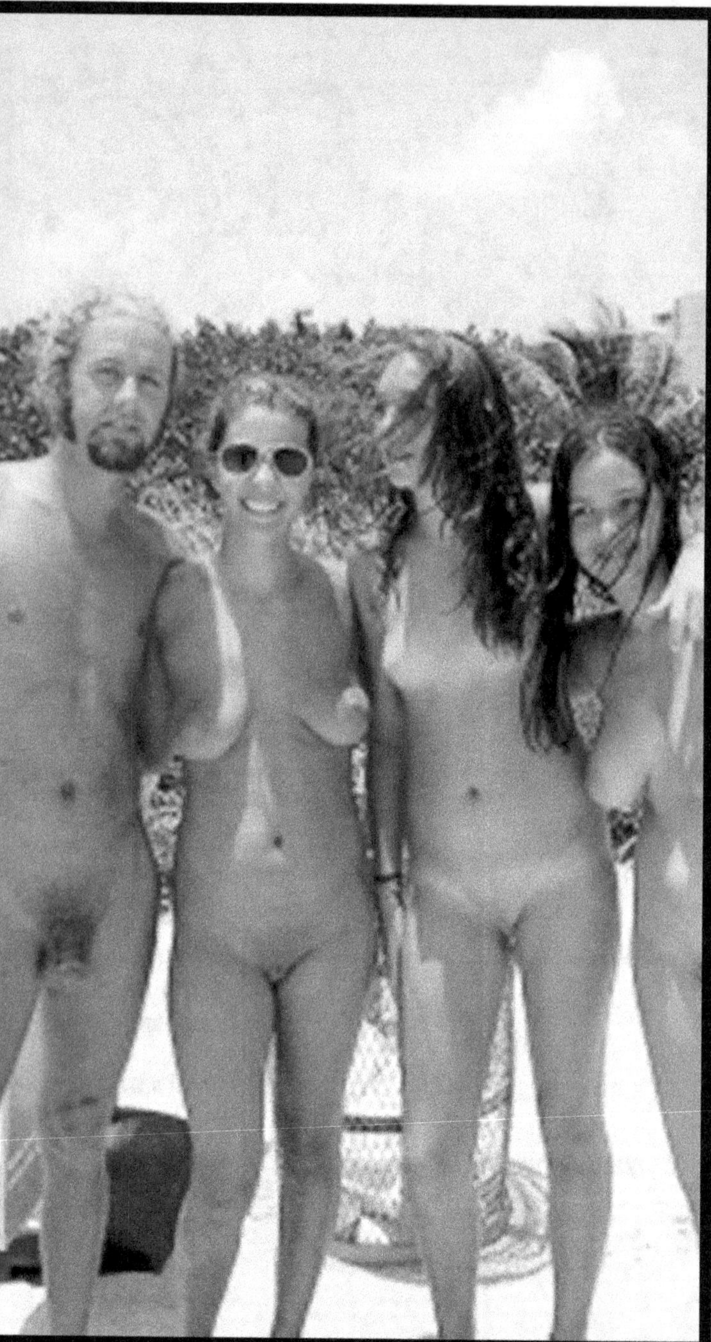

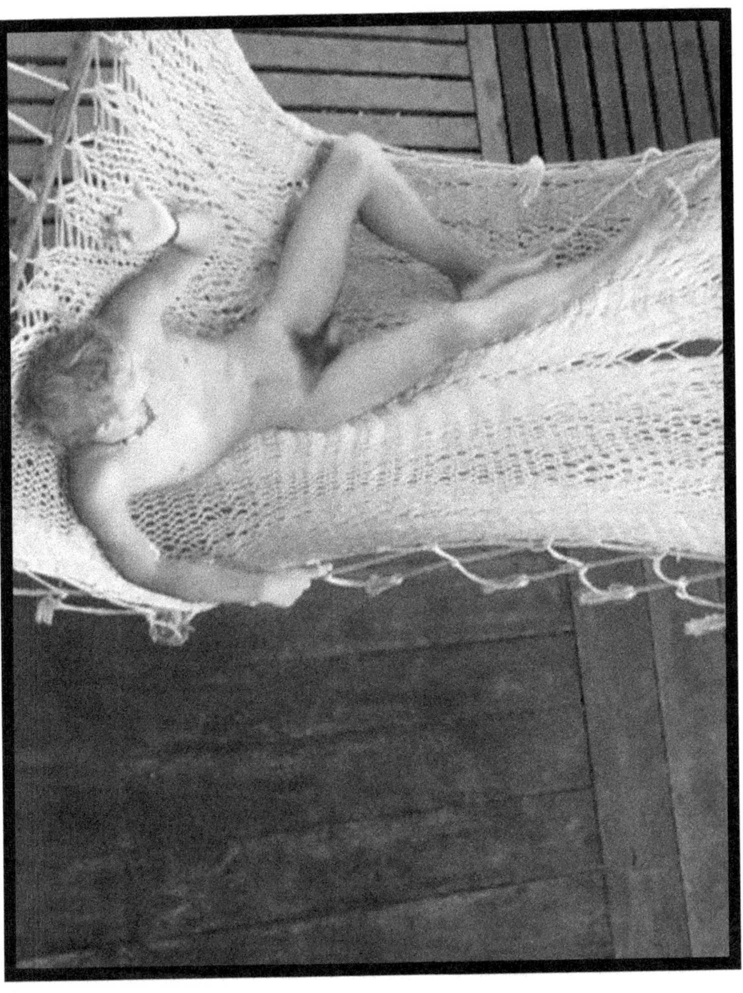

Better sleep, is a benefit as well. According to the National Sleep Foundation, in order to get an ideal level of restful sleep the body needs to be at an optimal temperature of 65 degrees, ditching clothes is the easiest, and most cost effective way of attaining that.

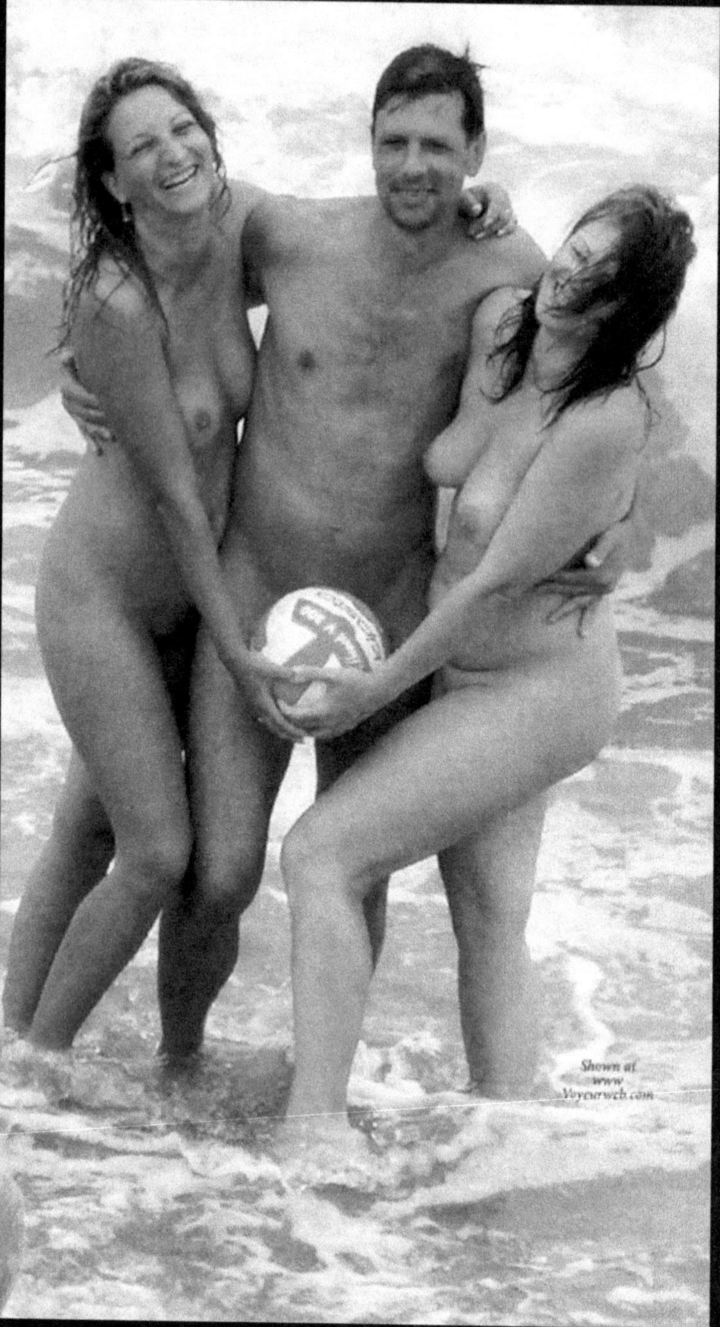
Shown at
www.
Voyeurweb.com

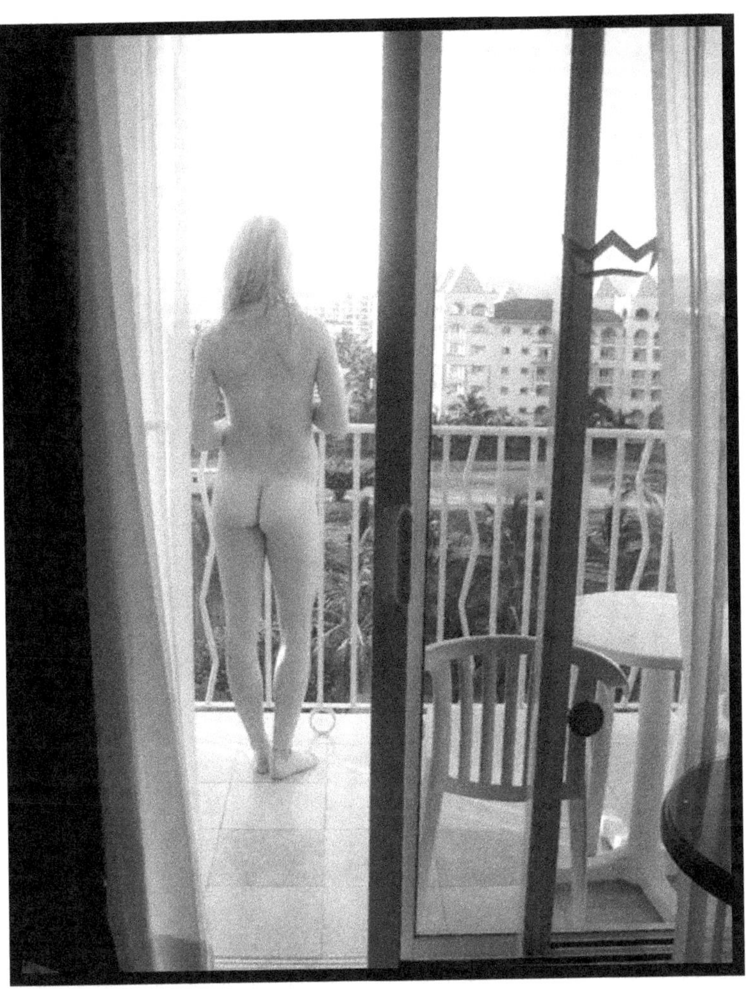

A lower body temperature has also shown to increase your metabolism and therefore boost weight loss. This means, becoming a nudist will help you lose weight.

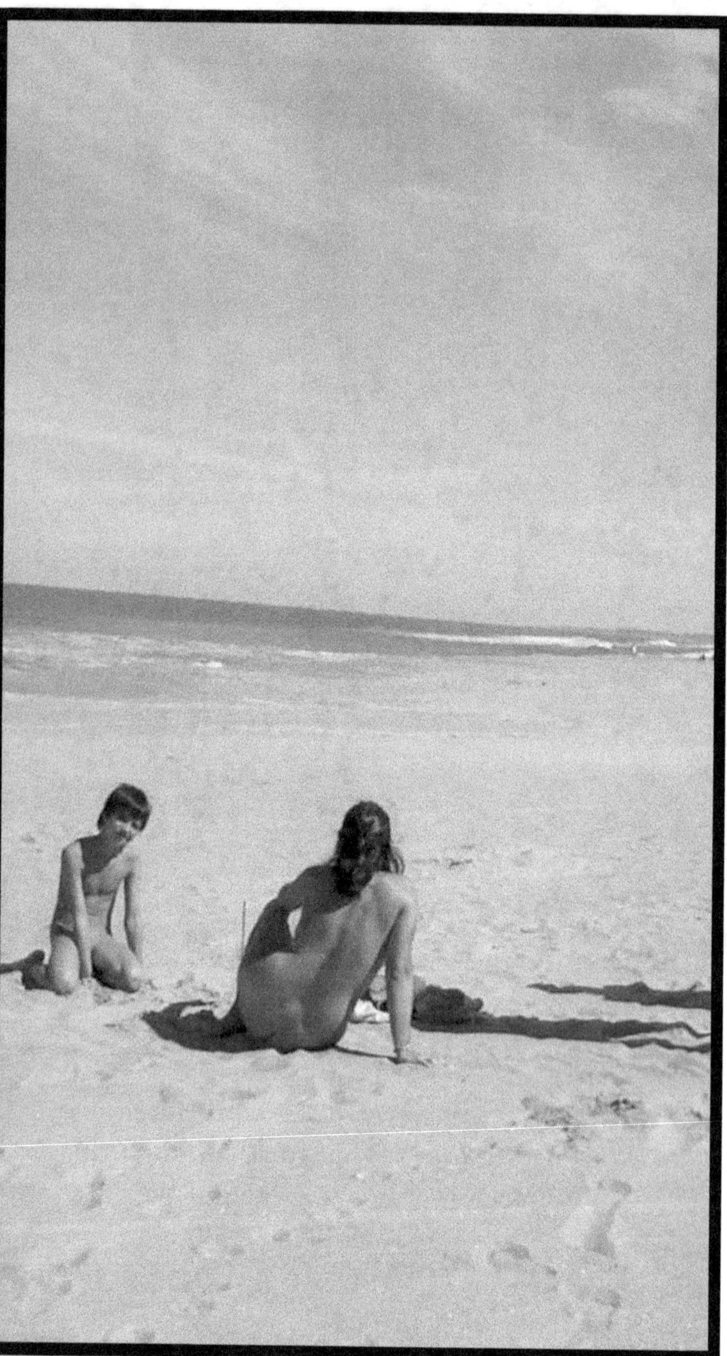

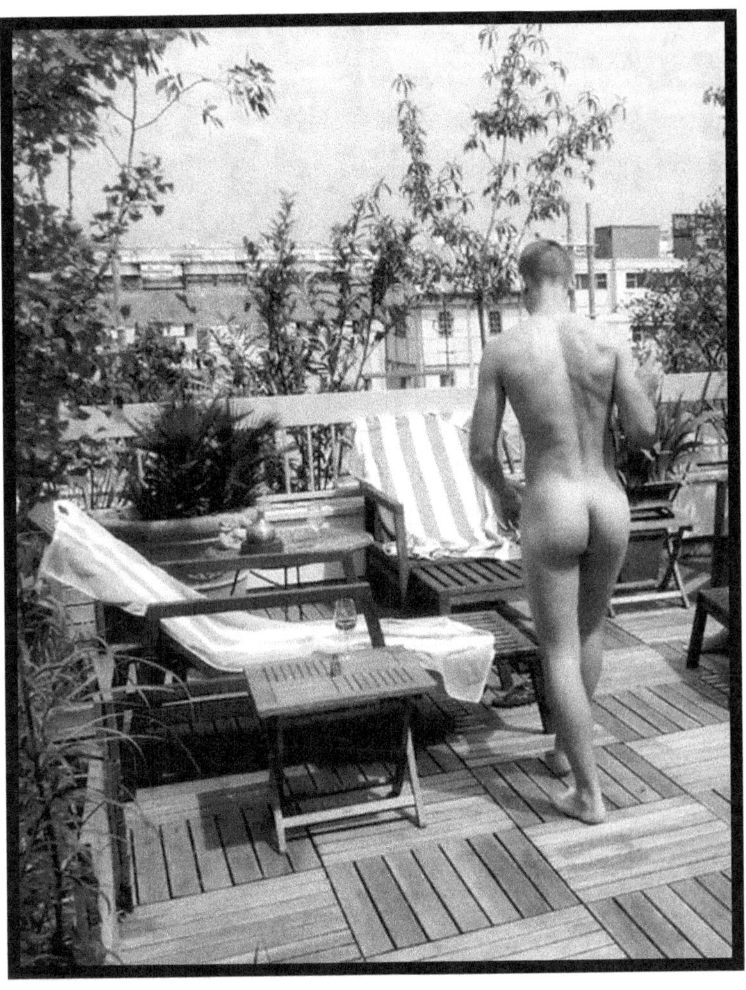

Doctor Michael Fiorillo, a plastic surgeon and skin care expert was quoted as saying, "Going naked is great for healthy skin. It helps the elimination of sweat toxins that clothing can reintroduce to the body and better overall blood circulation."

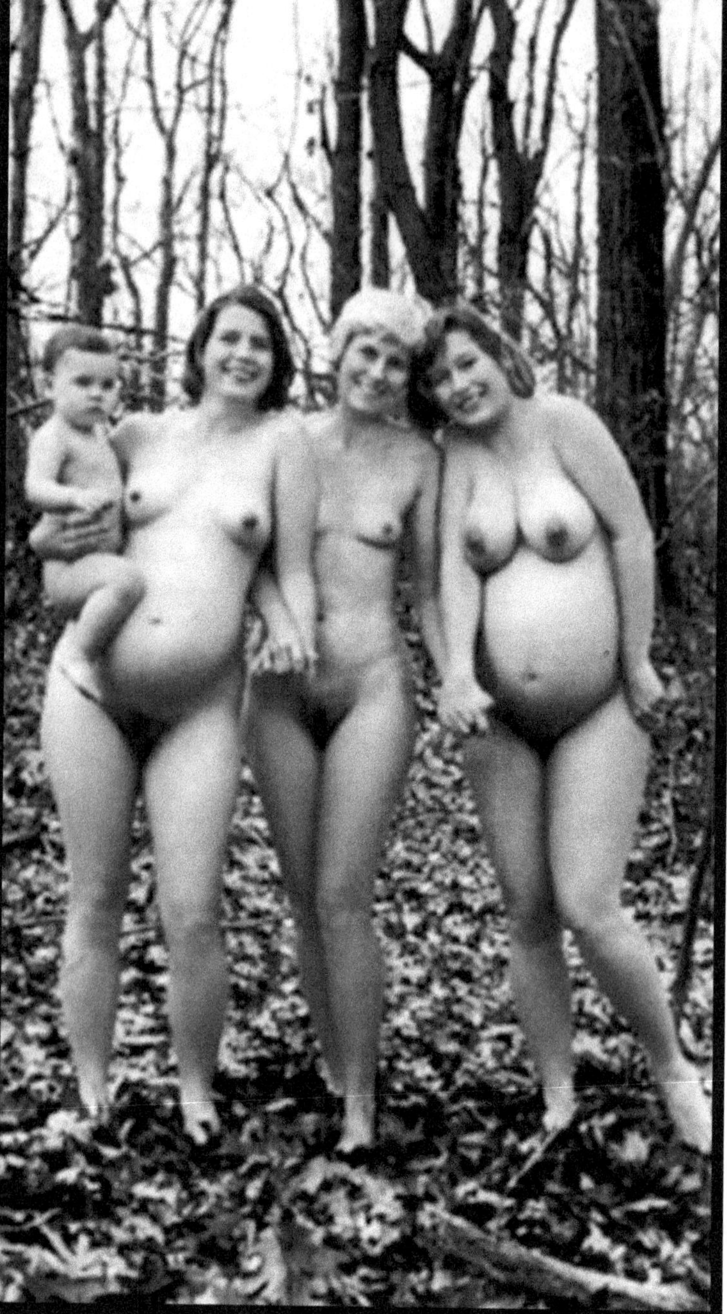

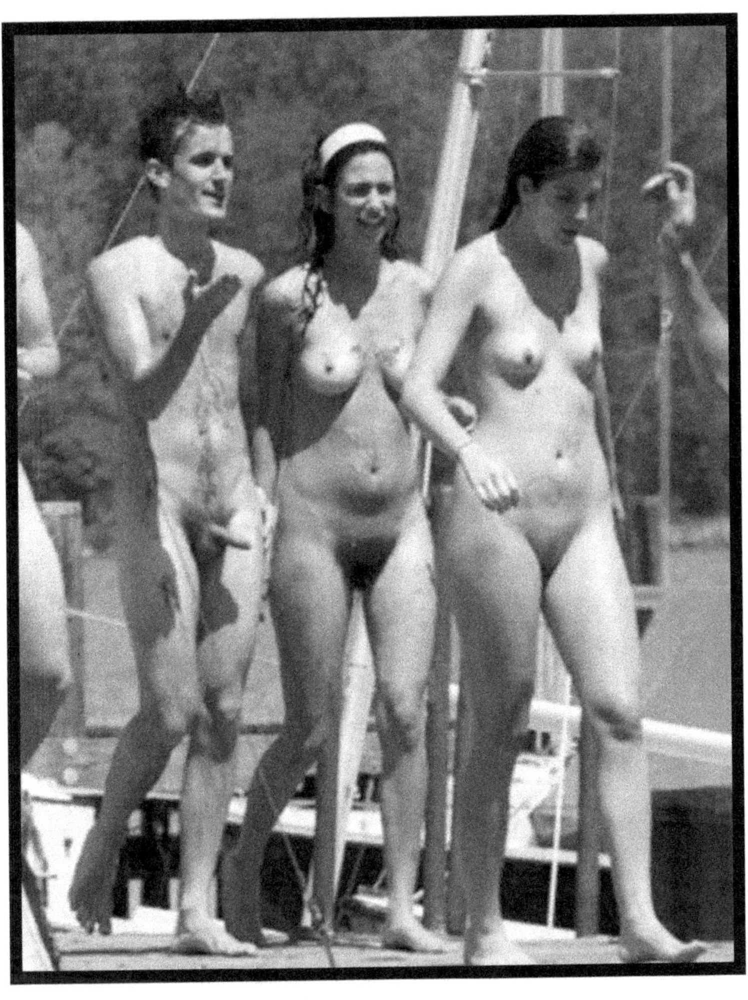

Doctor Lance Brown, a dermatologist in New York City, agreed, adding, "Wearing restrictive clothing can cause excessive sweating which may lead to inflammation of this skin follicles, rashes and breakouts. Going bare gives your skin a chance to breathe."

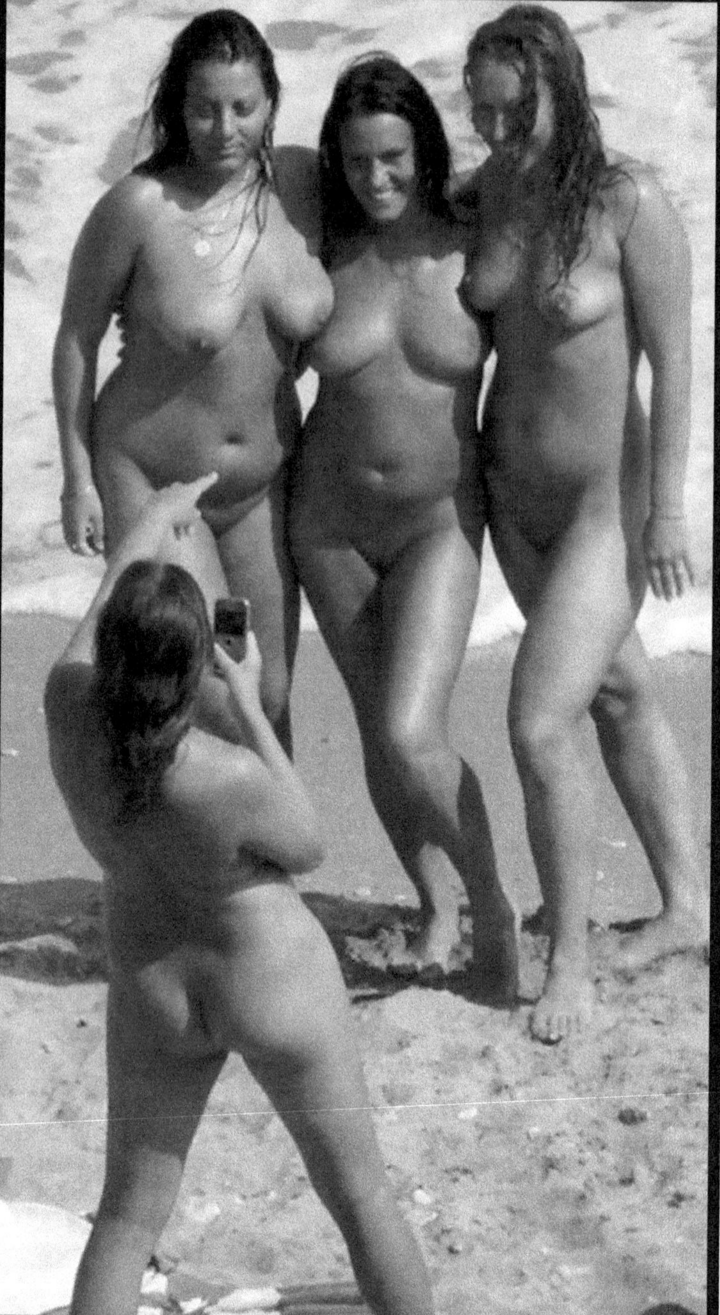

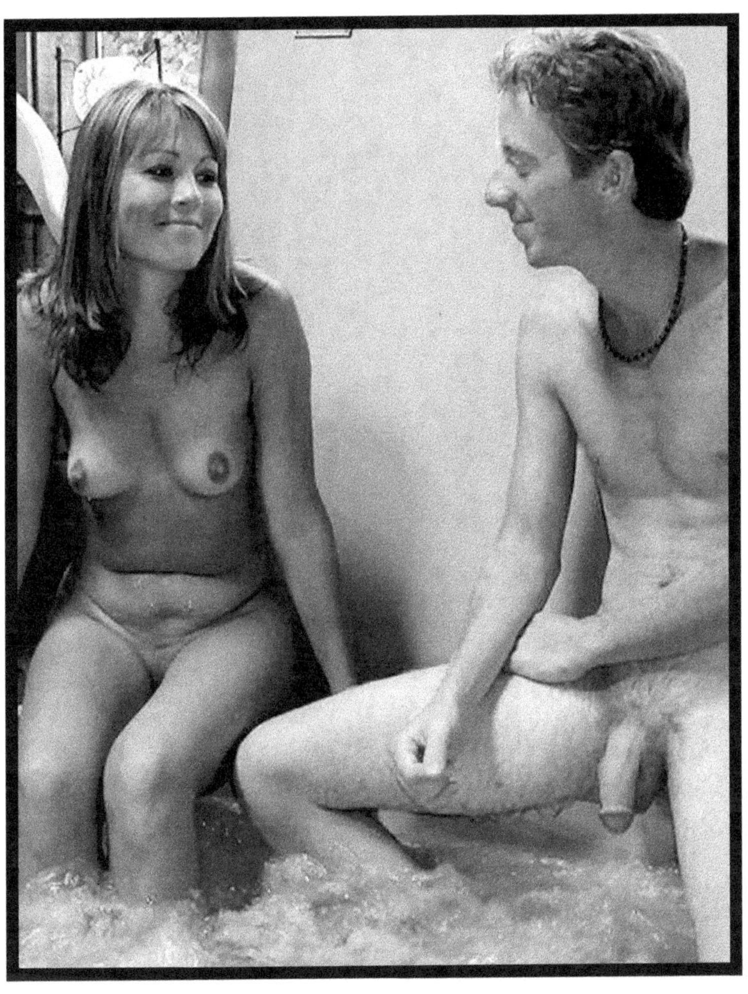

Relationship Expert Doctor Jenn Mann believes that more time in the buff can help men and women battle body image issues. "Spending time in the nude is a great way to get in touch with your body. Most people in today's society are so disconnected from bodily sensations, and this could help." She goes on to say, "Being in the nude reduces shame. You can work on self-acceptance and that can be very healing."

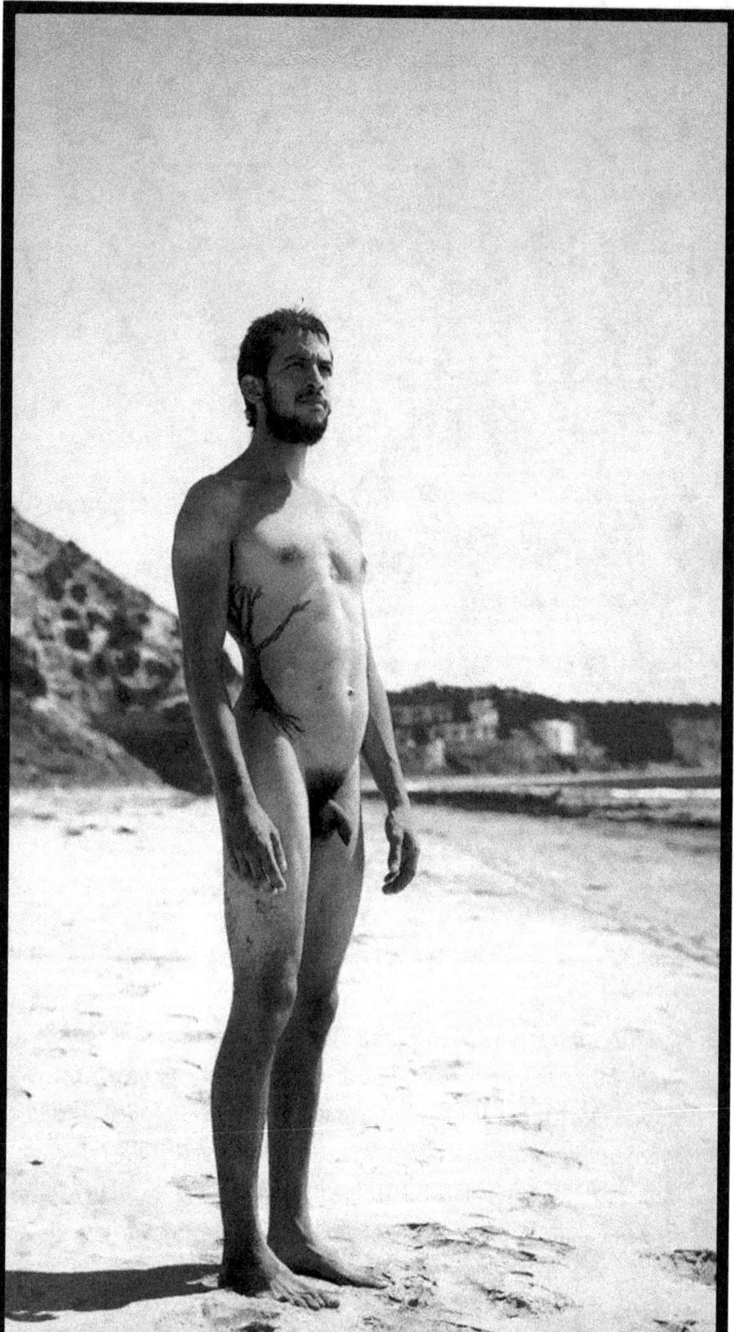

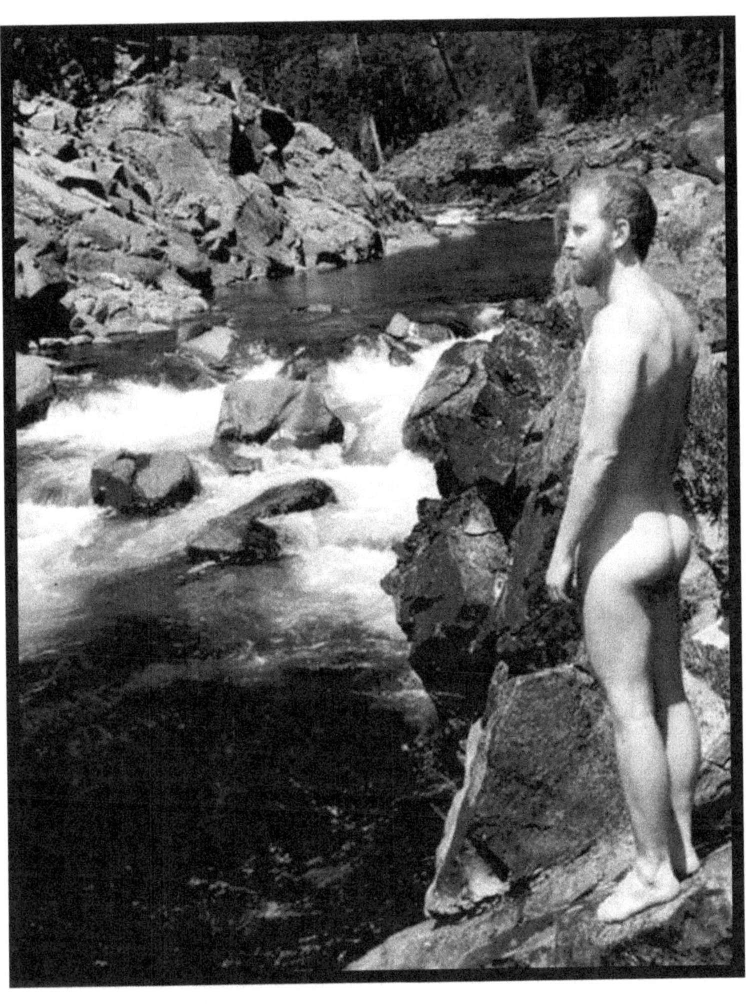

All of these doctors and experts are explaining the benefits from a medical standpoint. But in my opinion, the self-esteem boosting effect is probably the most important thing.

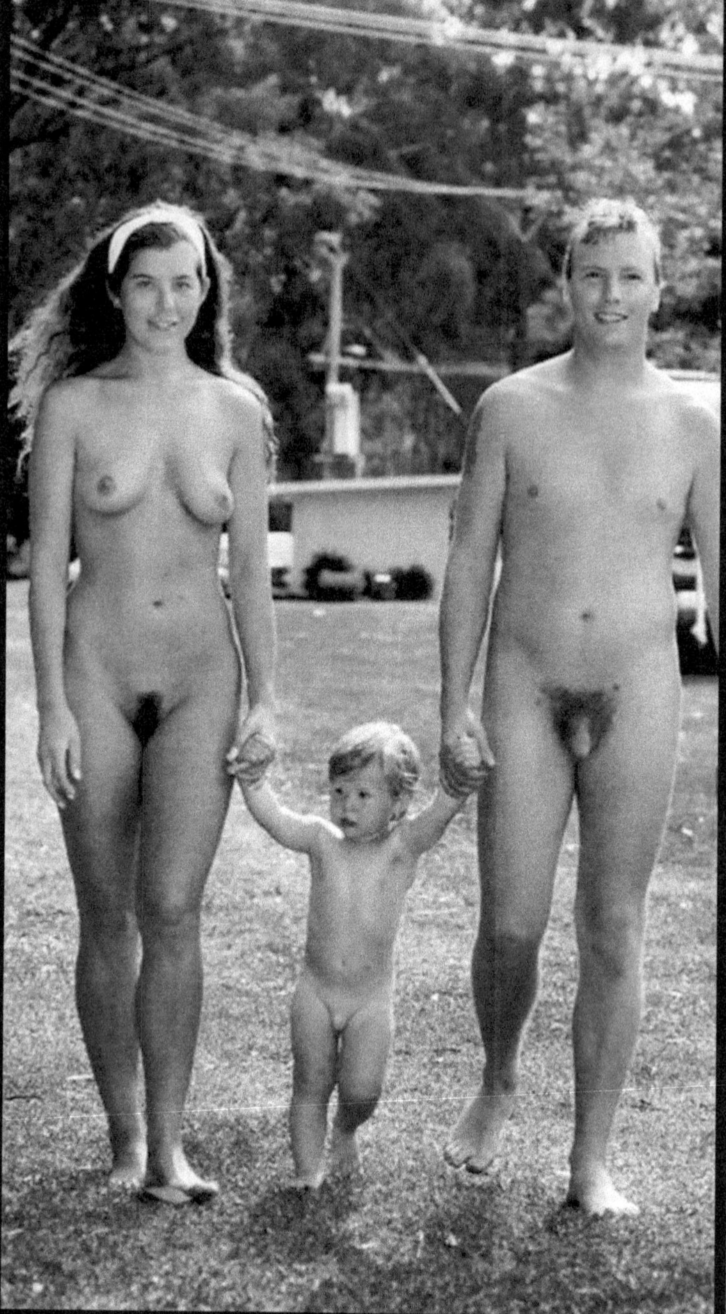

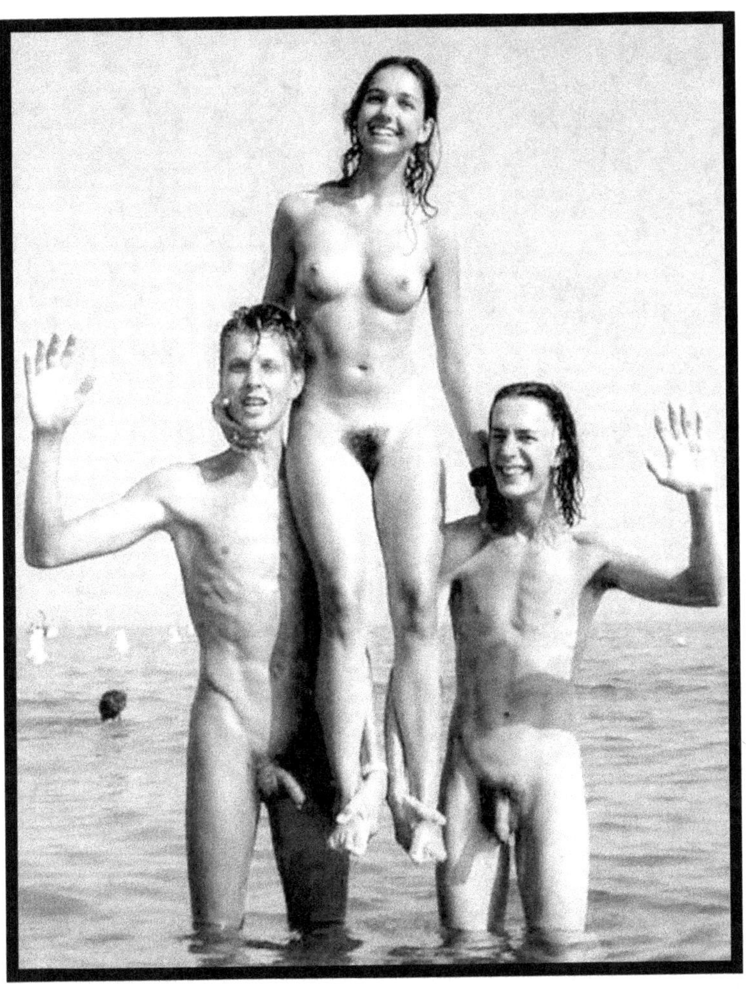

By practicing nudism in groups or social settings, you learn to let go of inhibitions and just go with the flow, seeing that others are not fazed by nudity helped me personally embrace it.

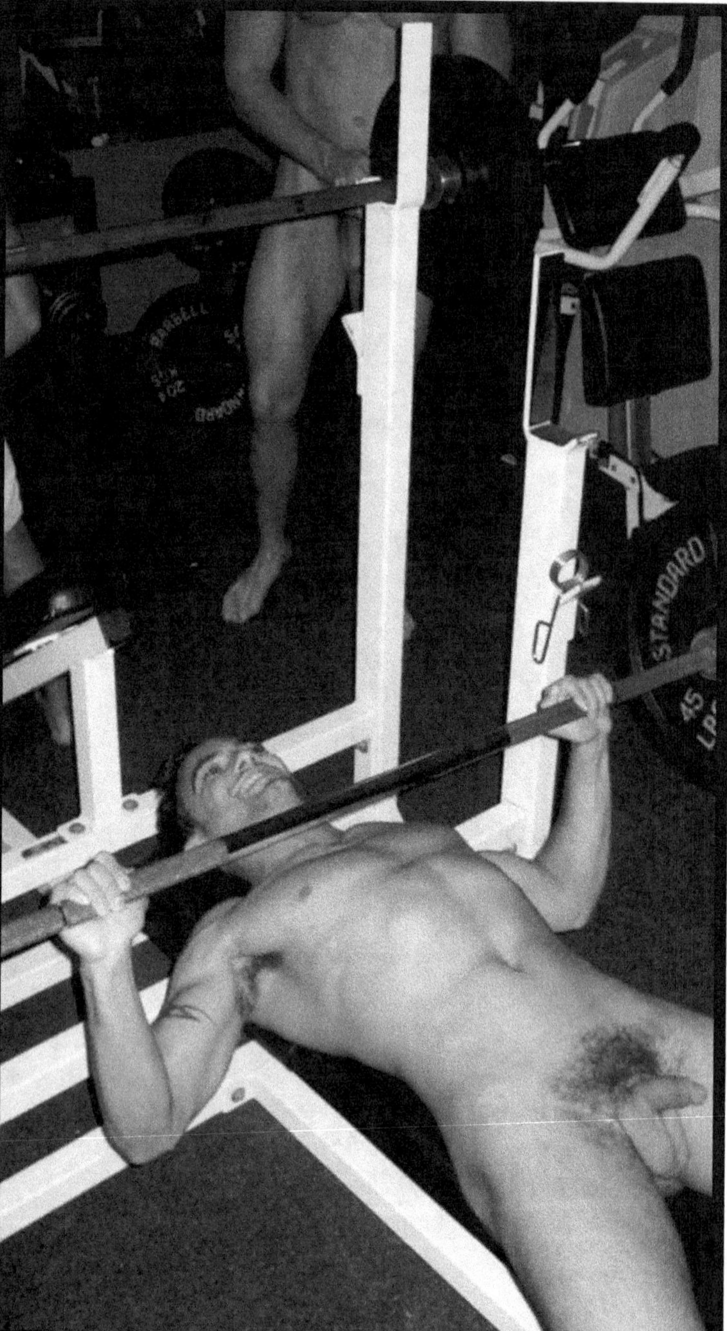

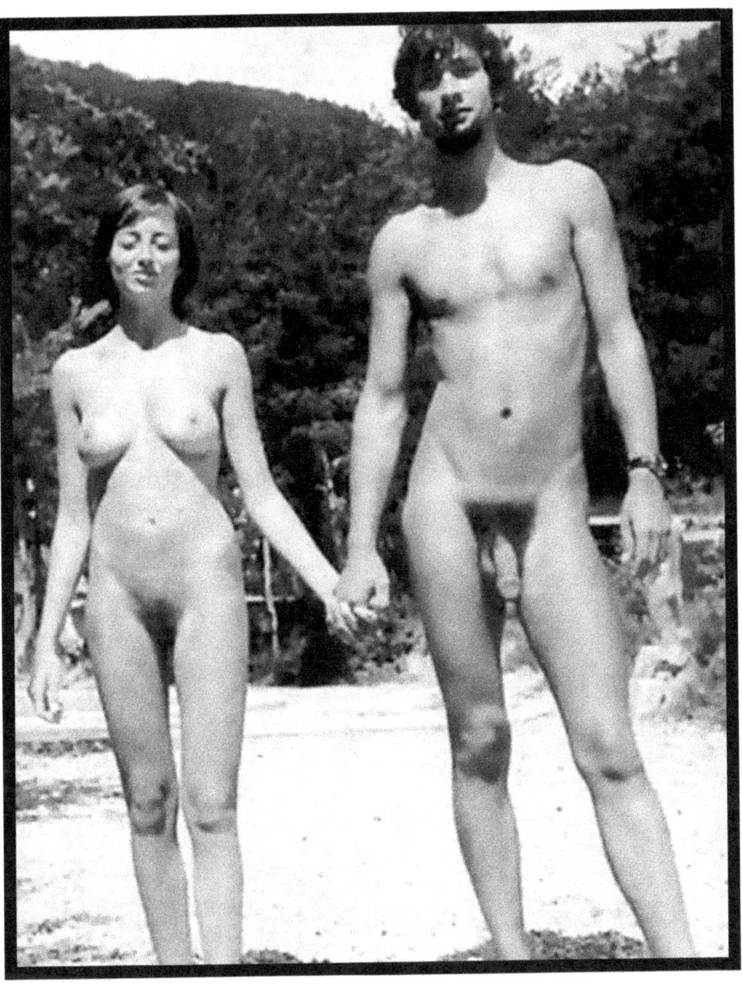

Living the Nudist Life is a great thing to do as a family, and has tremendous self-esteem building effects on kids and teens, but I will go into that in a later section.

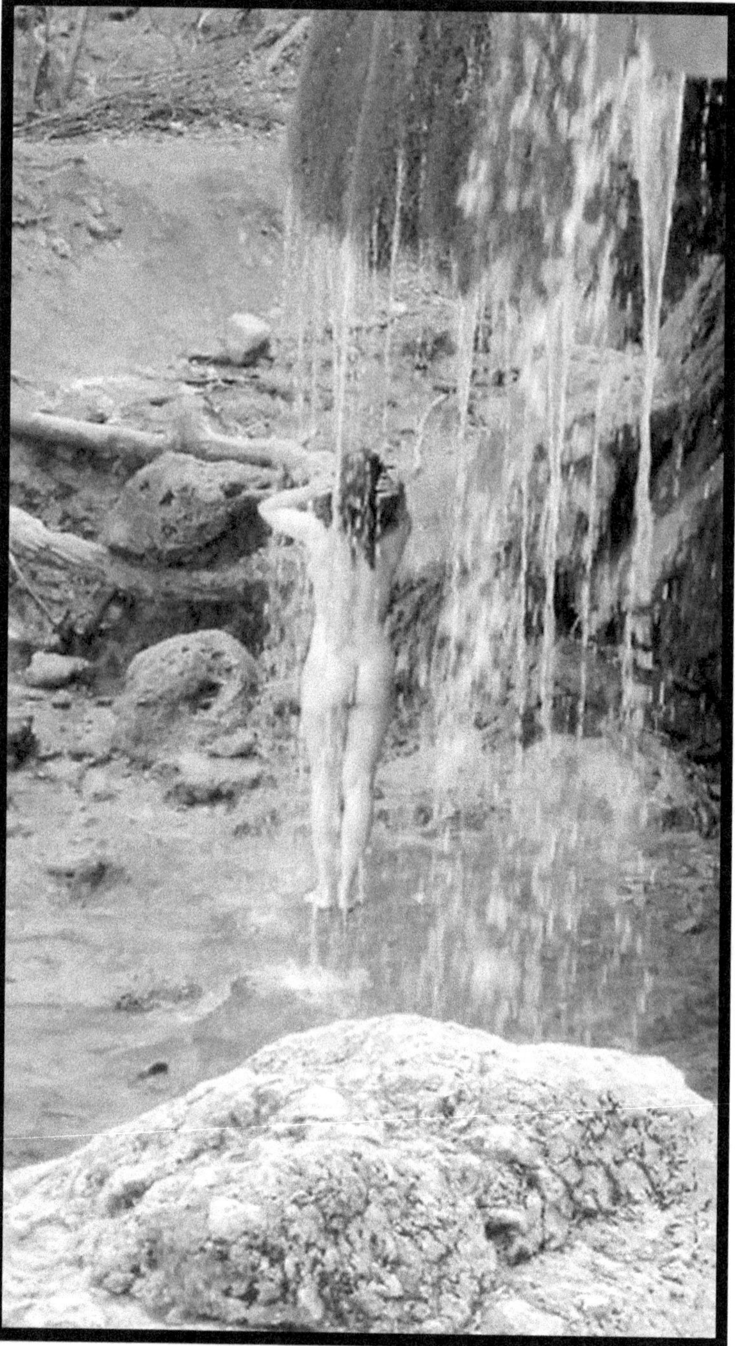

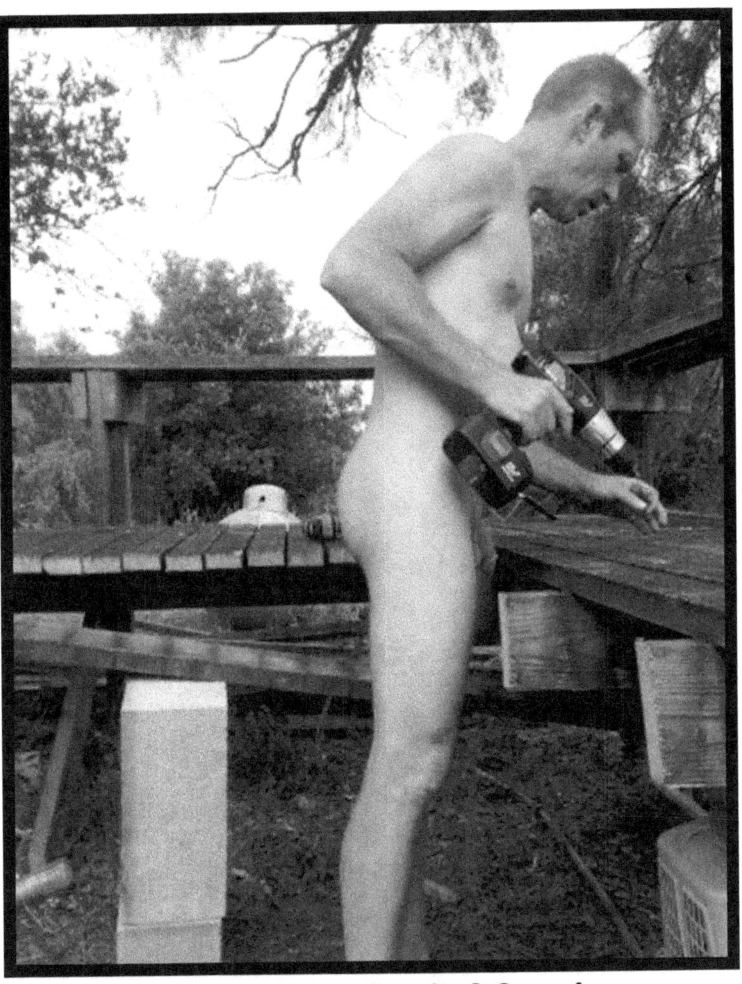

Nudism in a Social Setting

Nudism is a great thing to do on your own, and there should never be any pressure to embrace it outside of your comfort zone. However, socializing with other nudists can be an amazing experience, and in my opinion is crucial to being able to appreciate the full benefits of nudism.

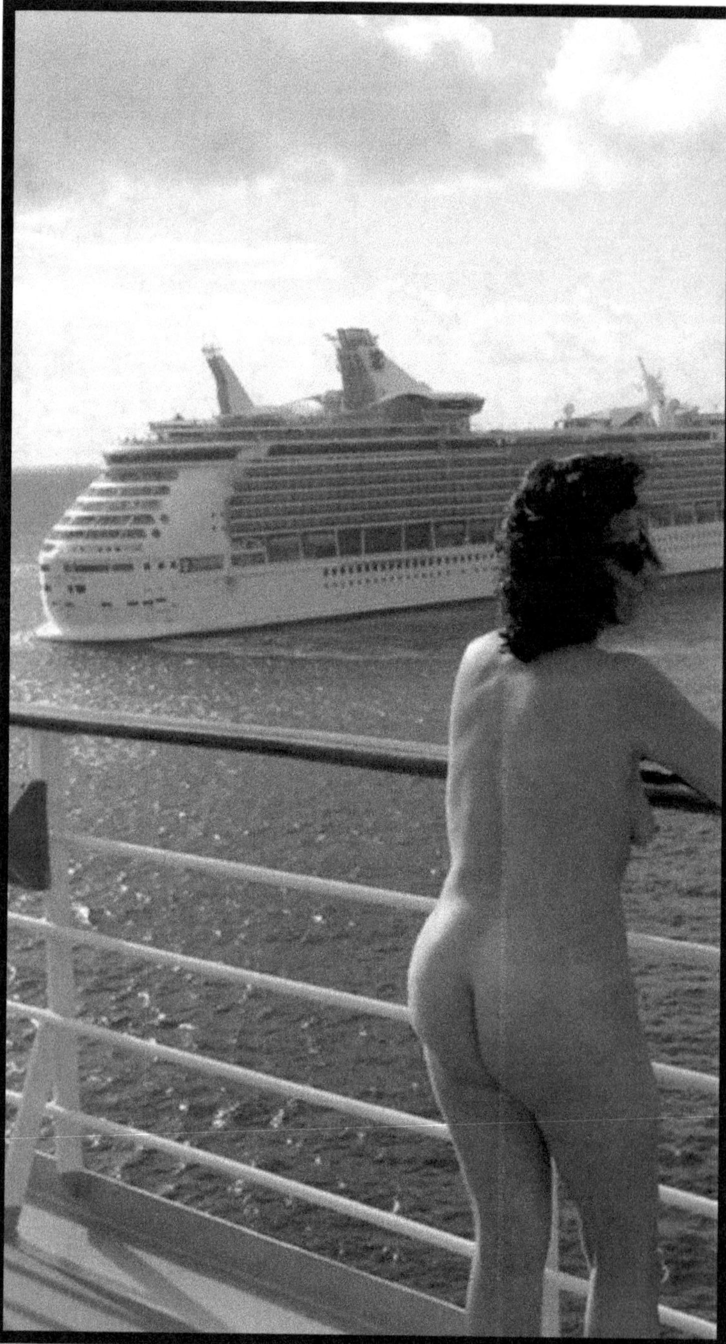

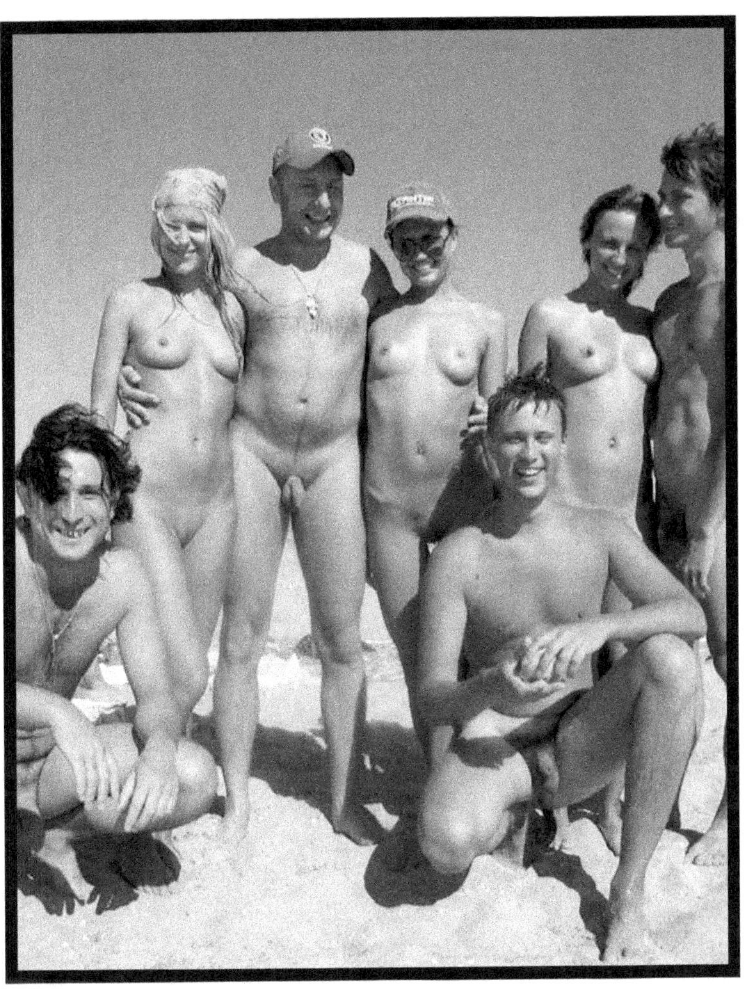

There are many ways to engage in social nudism, from nude beaches, to spas, to resorts. One of the most popular locations in my area is Gunnison Beach, in New Jersey. In 1999 the state of New Jersey essentially made it illegal to be nude on state beaches, however Gunnison is on Federal Land, so those laws do not apply.

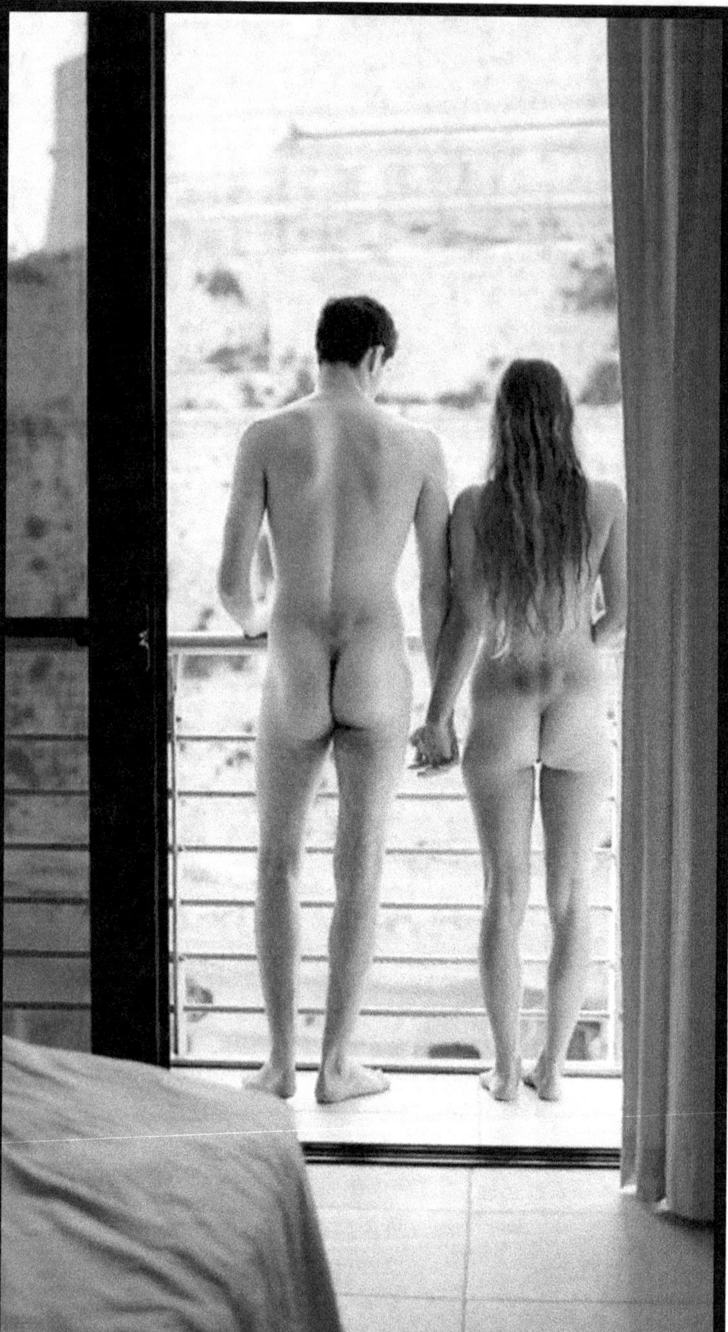

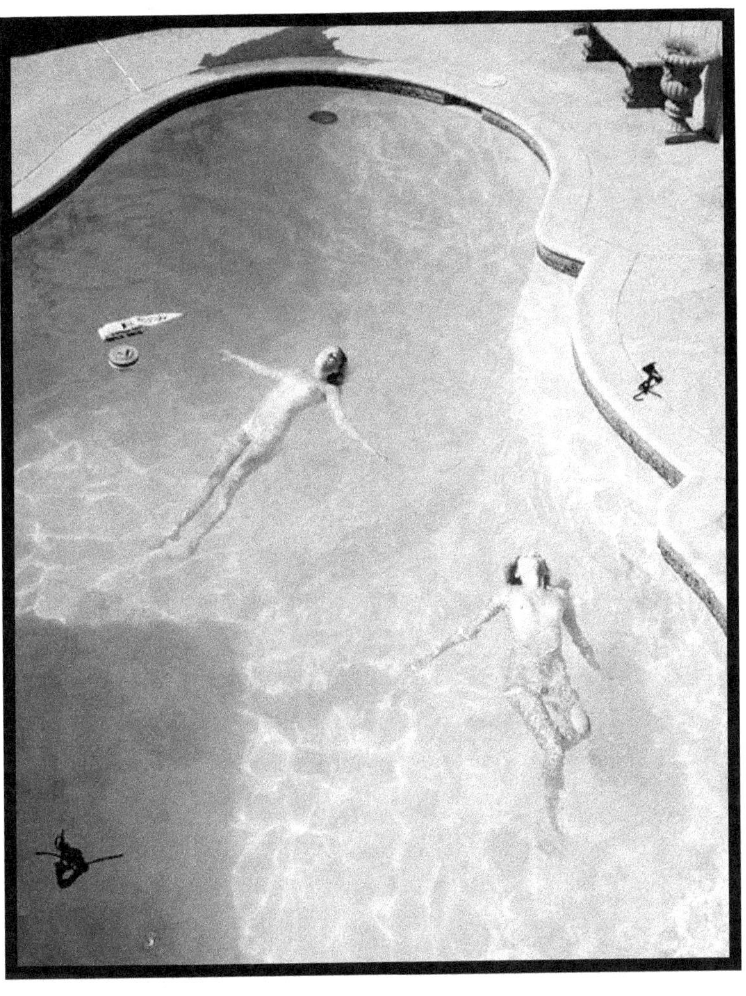

If you have never had a chance to skinny dip or go to a nude beach, I highly recommend giving it a try. While people compare skinny dipping in a pool to taking a bath, it really is a totally different sensation.

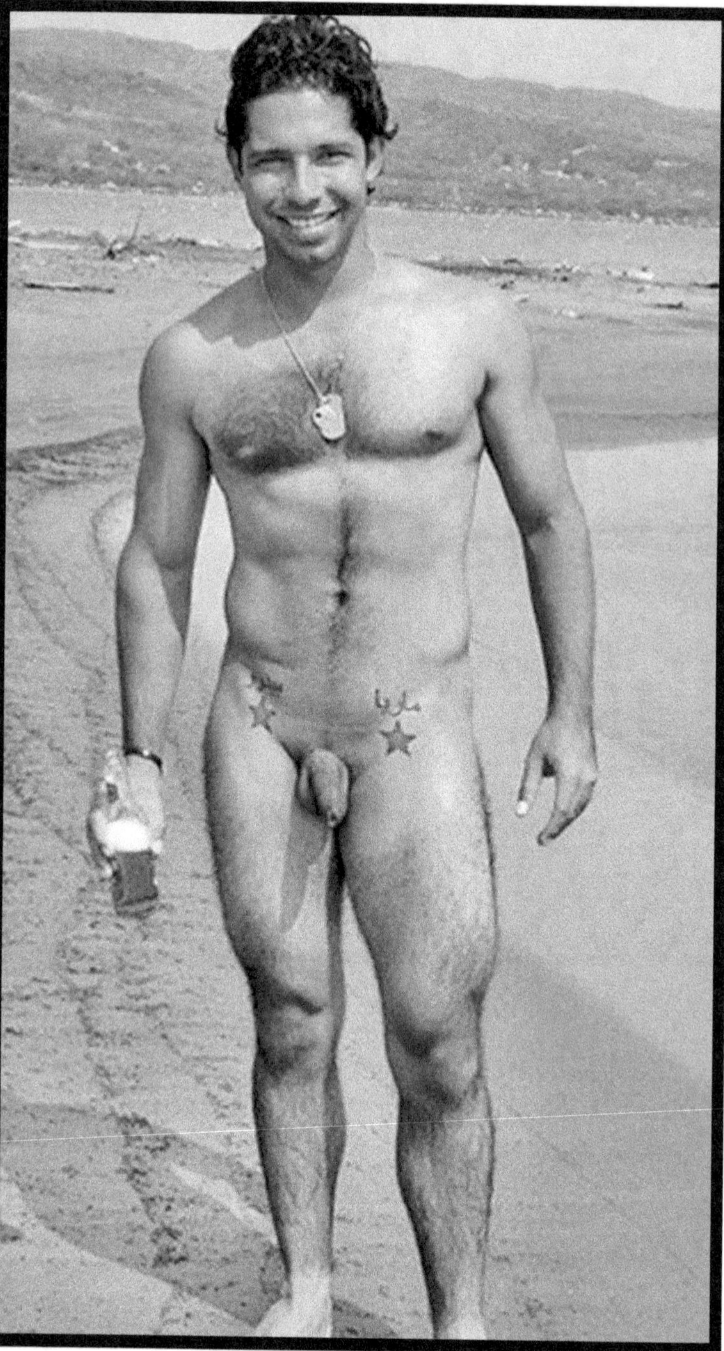

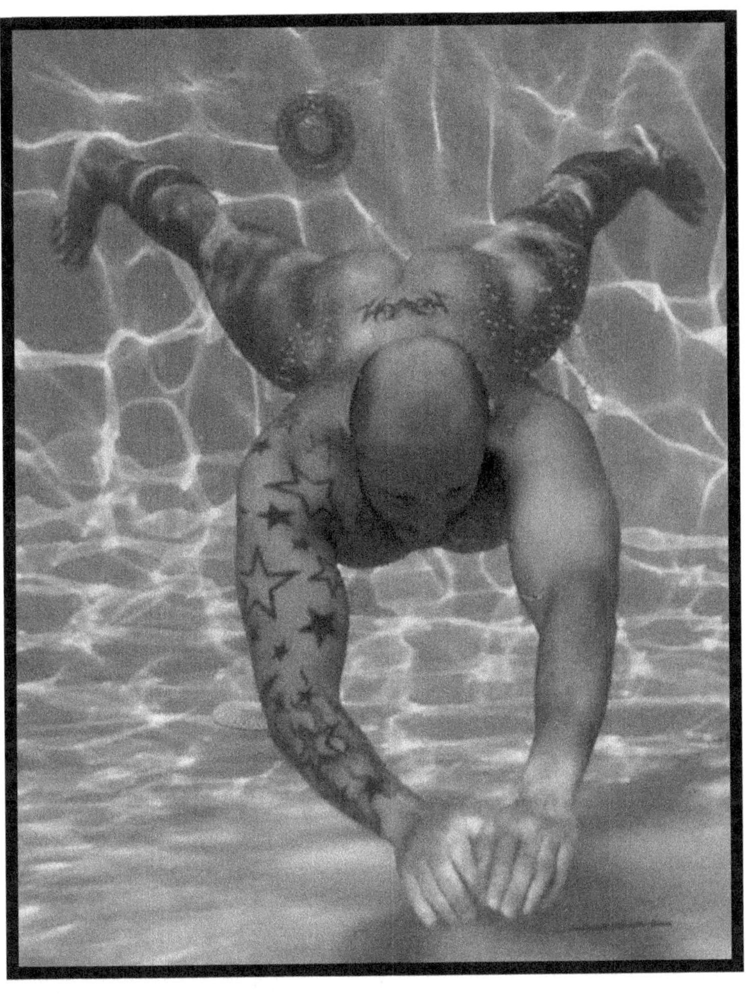

For the majority of my life, whenever I have gone swimming, I have worn a swimsuit. As a man, our swim trunks hold our male genital in place, similar to underwear. The first time I was in a pool and took off my swimsuit, let me just say it was a life changing moment.

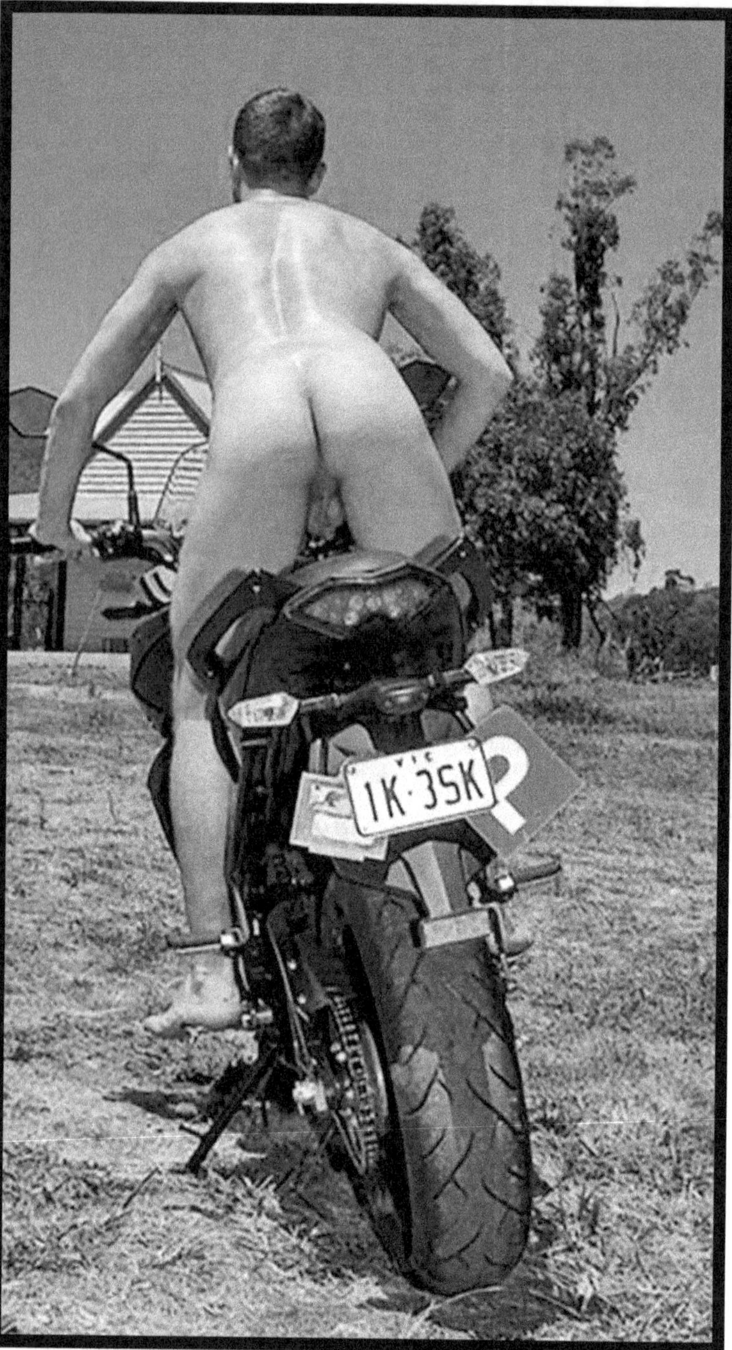

VIC
1K·3SK

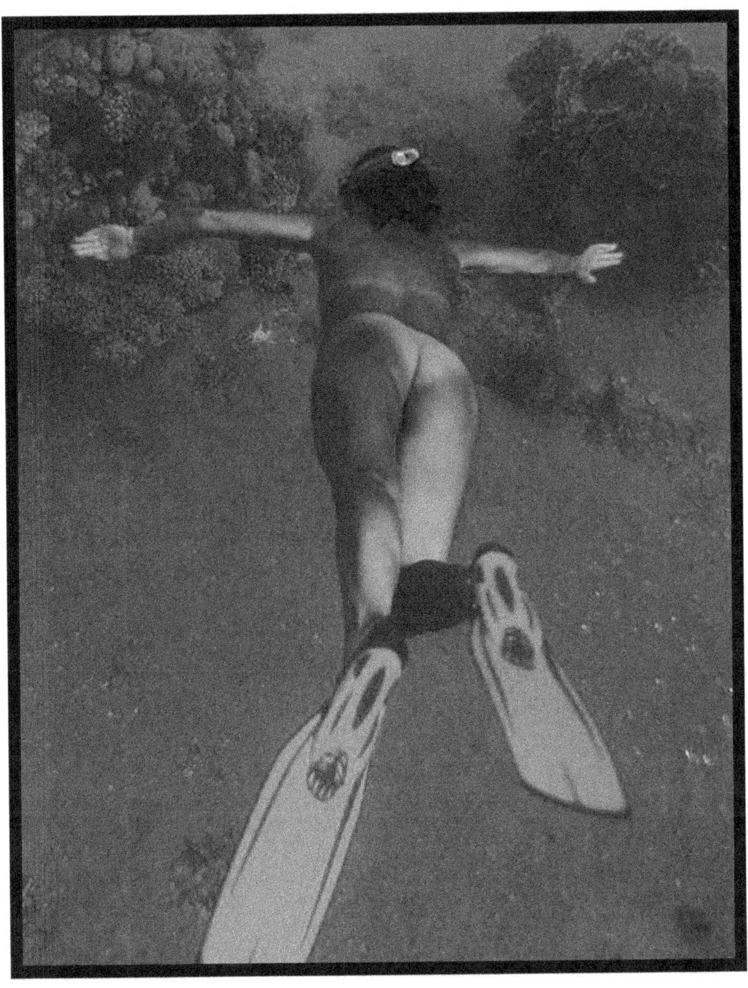

Similar to the free feeling of walking around your house nude, the free feeling is amplified underwater, where usually your genitals would be held in by the swim trunks, they are allowed to move freely. It is the same for a woman who has never swam topless, and tries it for the first time. While this is amazing in itself, the experience of a pool is totally different from a beach.

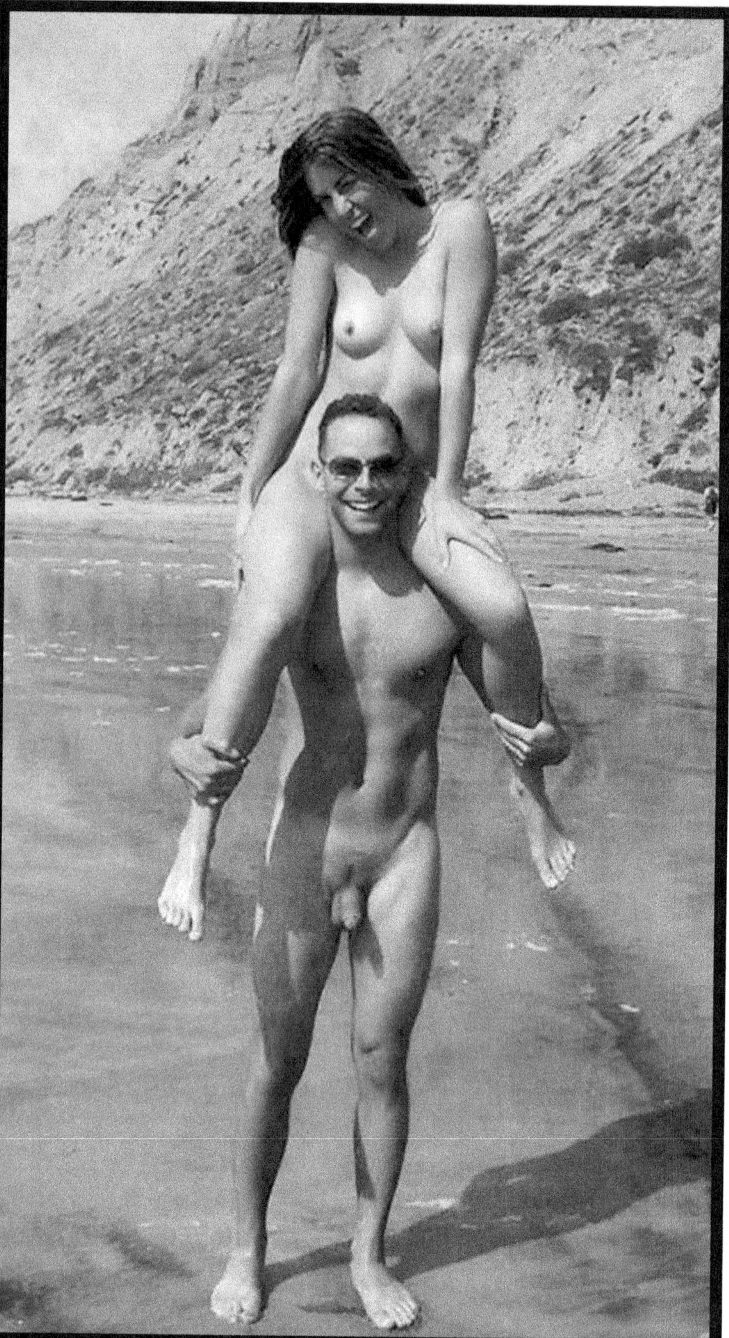

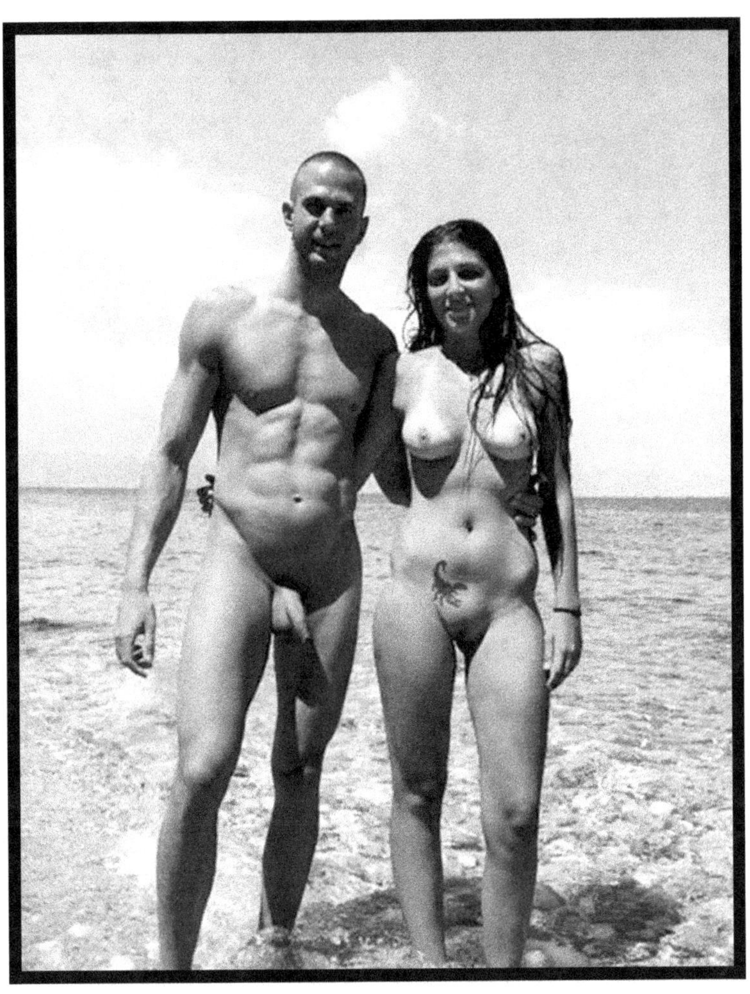

Being able to lie on the sand, allowing parts of your body, which have never seen the light of day, to be exposed to sand, sun and surf, is a truly enlightening feeling. Feeling the warm sand against your body, or feeing the movement of the waves brush against you, and the salty air breeze.

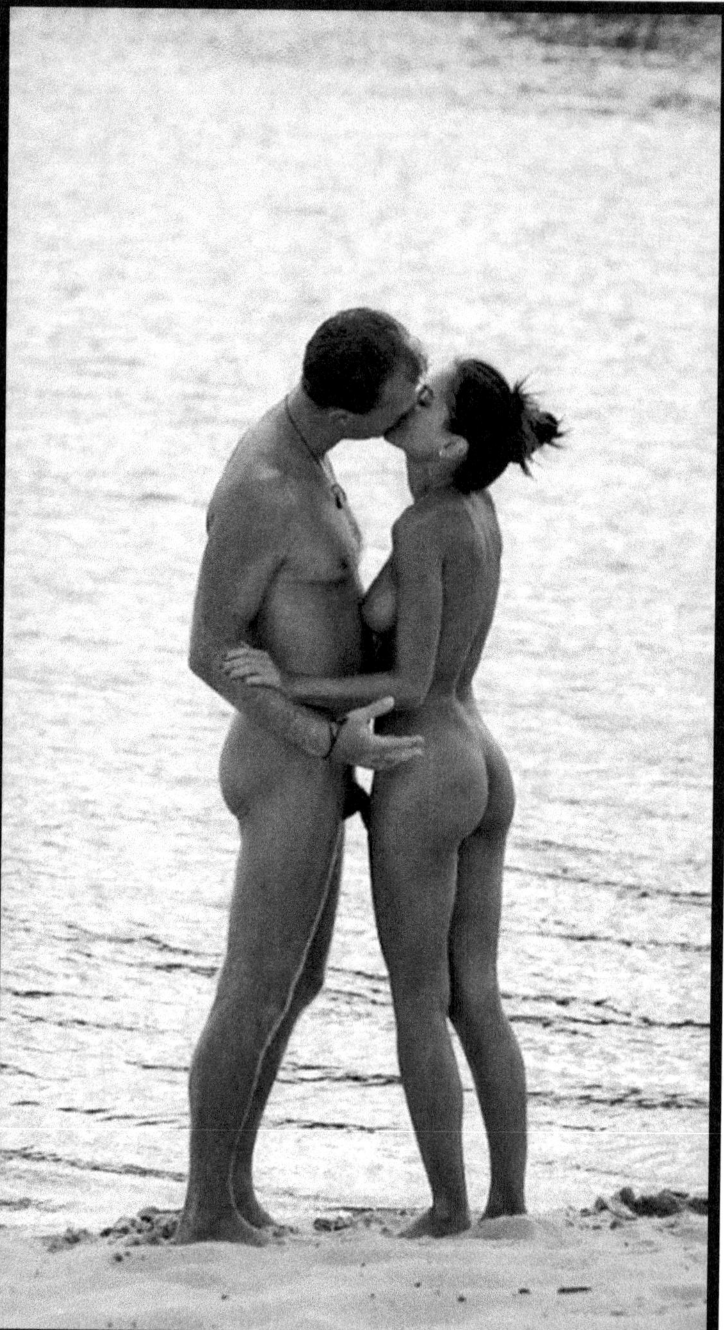

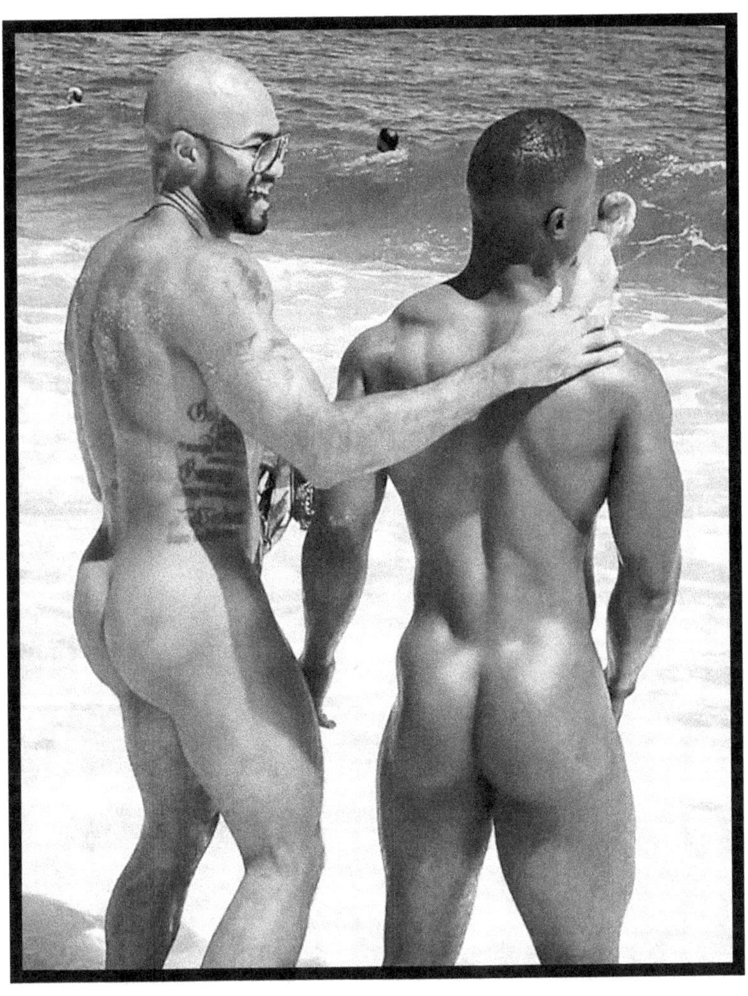

While no one wants to get sand in their nether regions, it's no different than getting sand in your hair, simply rinse it off and there are no issues.

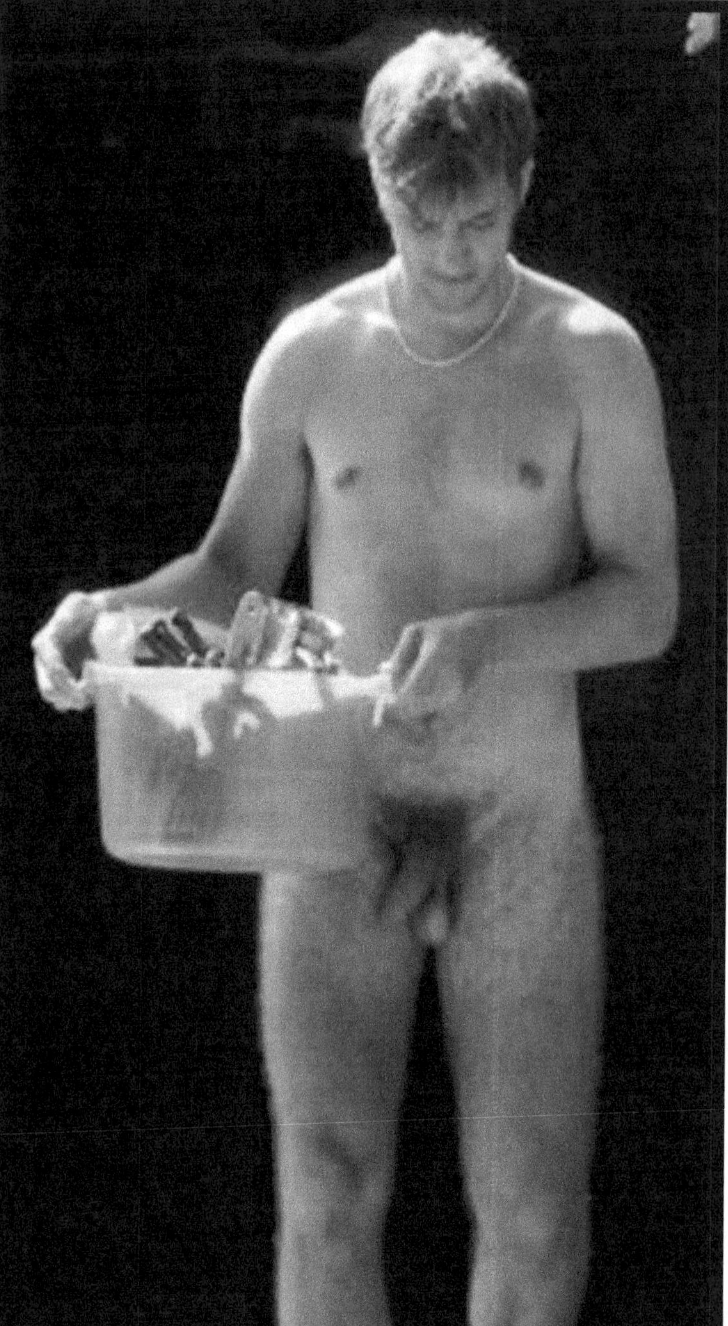

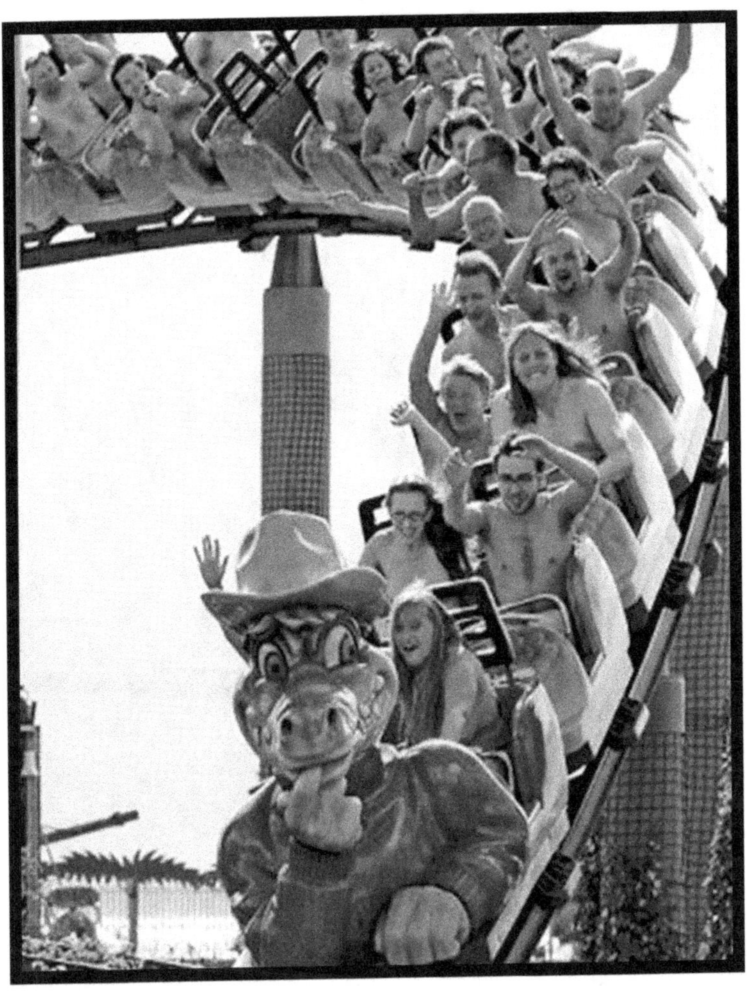

Like I mentioned earlier though, pool and beaches aren't the only social thing one can embrace. There are nudist resorts all over this country, and all over the world, where nudists can meet other nudists, relax on the beach and partake in sports.

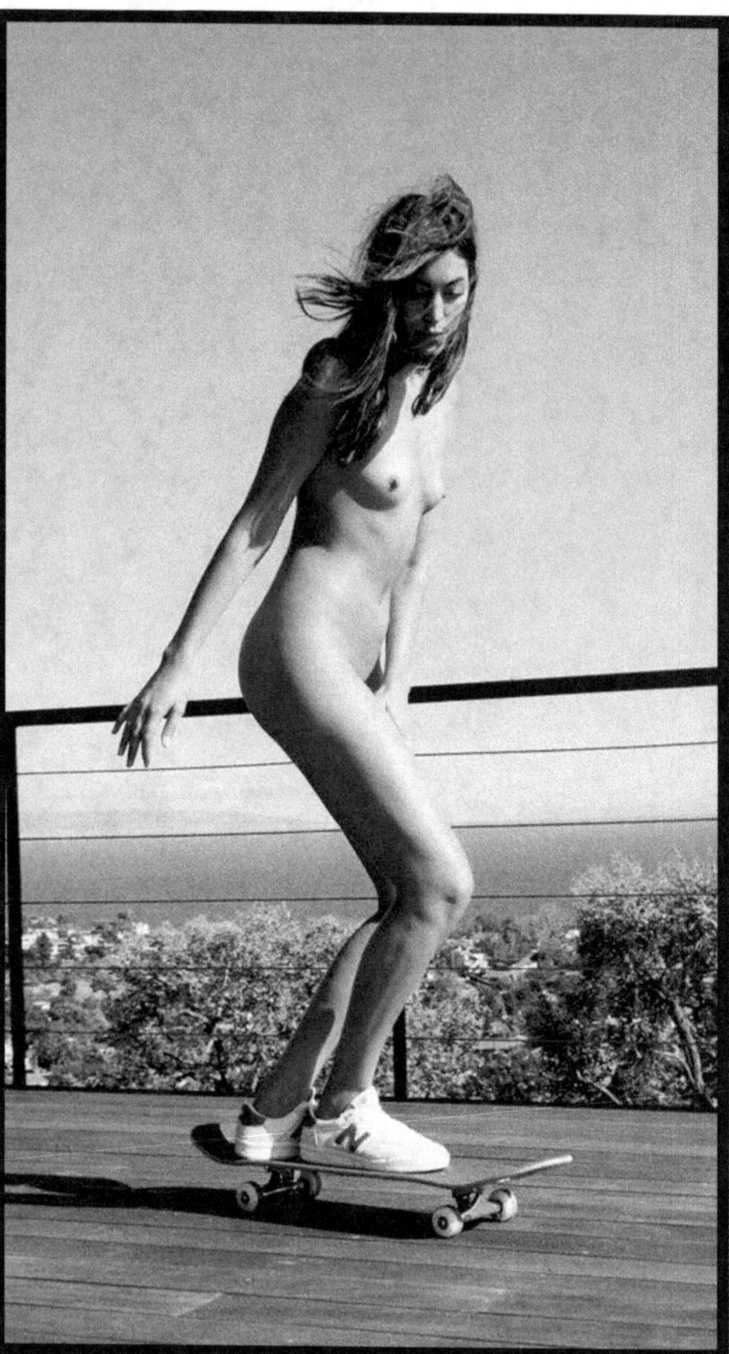

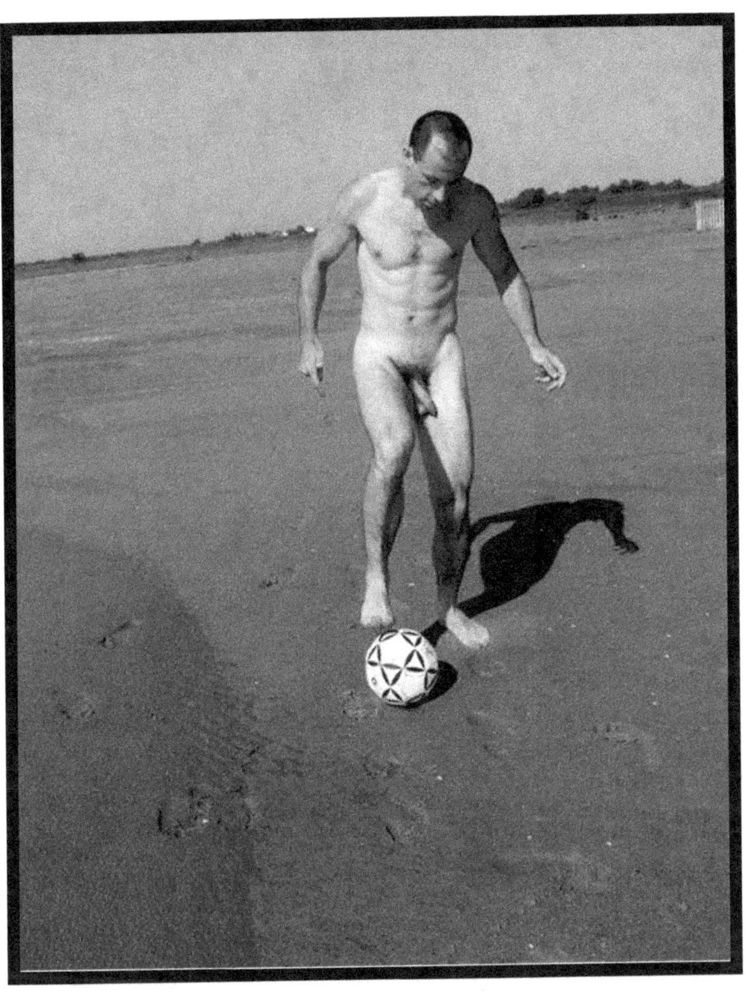

Nude soccer and volleyball are very popular pastimes for both adults and kids of all ages. Of course, it's played the same as of you were wearing clothes, it is still the same game. Getting into a nude sport will help with removing inhibition, since you tend to be focused on the game instead of what other people are thinking.

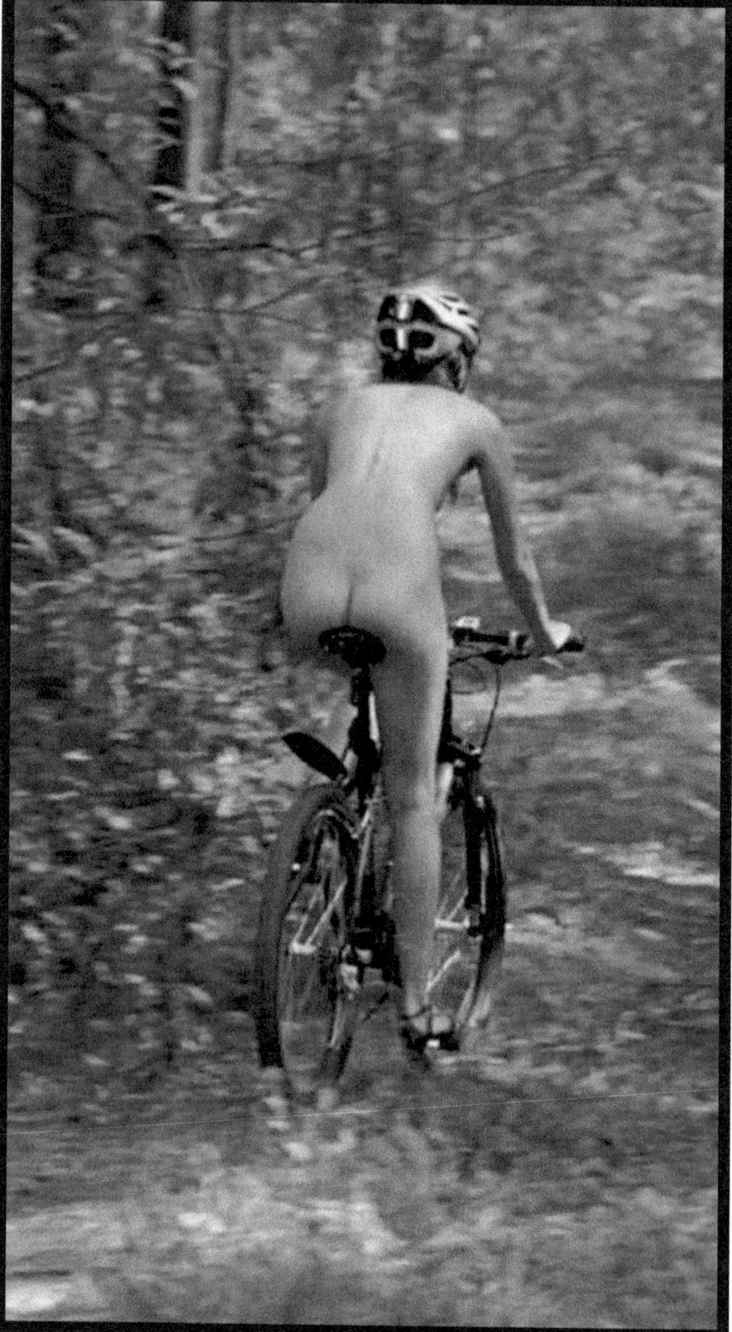

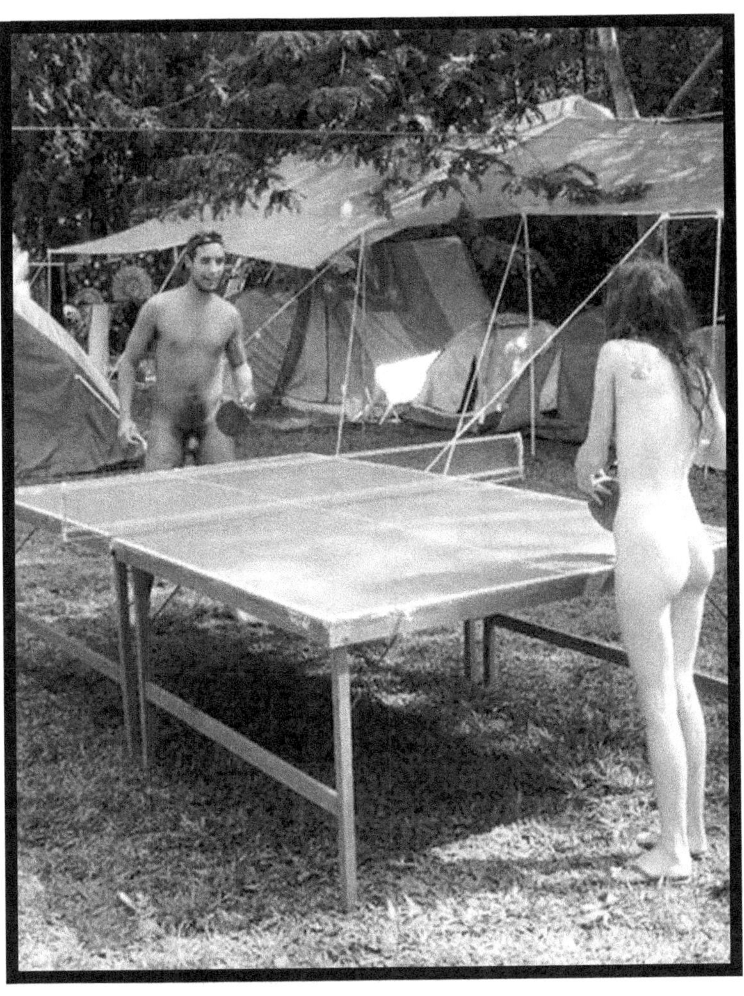

Just like Nude Resorts, there are Nude Cruises, and several cruise lines offer nude cruises throughout the year. This is just another way for nudists to congregate and meet others of like mind, in a social environment where everyone can feel comfortable.

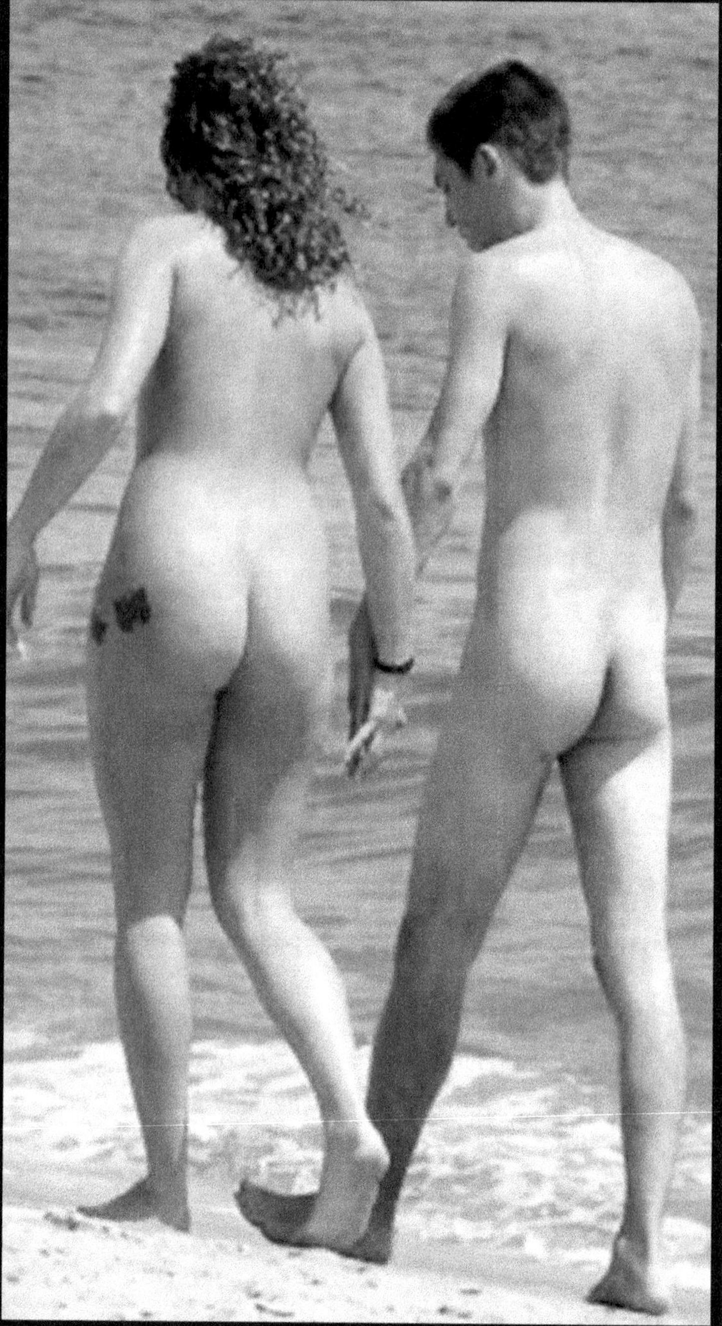

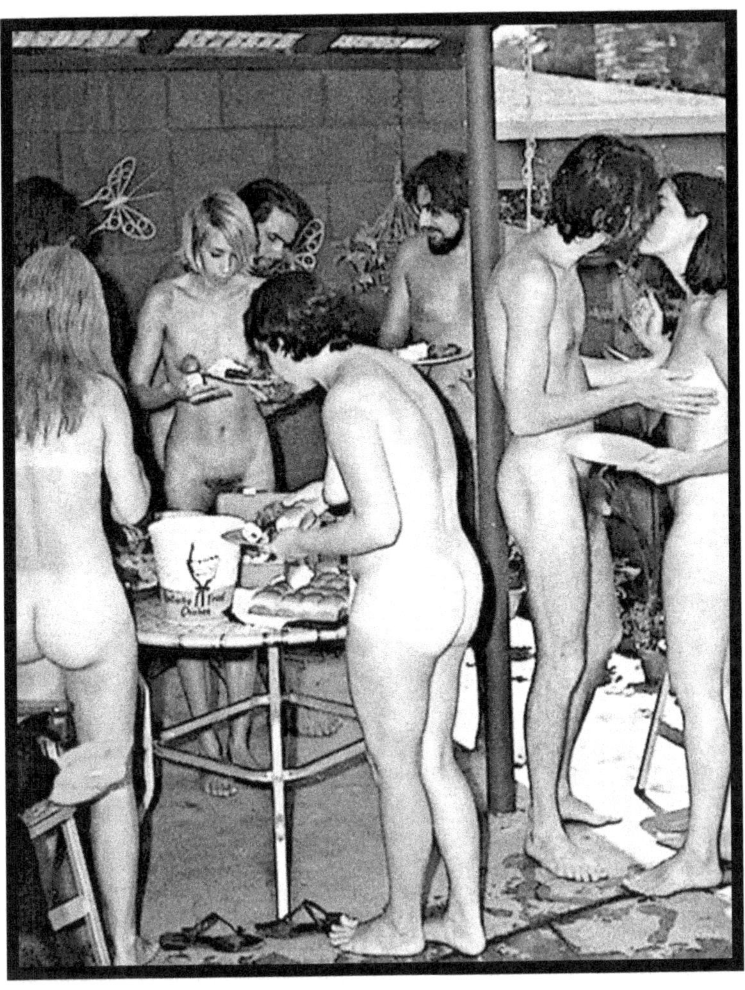

One thing that I particularly love, is hosting or attending a nudist dinner party or game night. It's so simple, have a glass of wine, dinner, and play some board games or whatever. Like any dinner party, it's just an informal way to relax and embrace social nudism with the company of others.

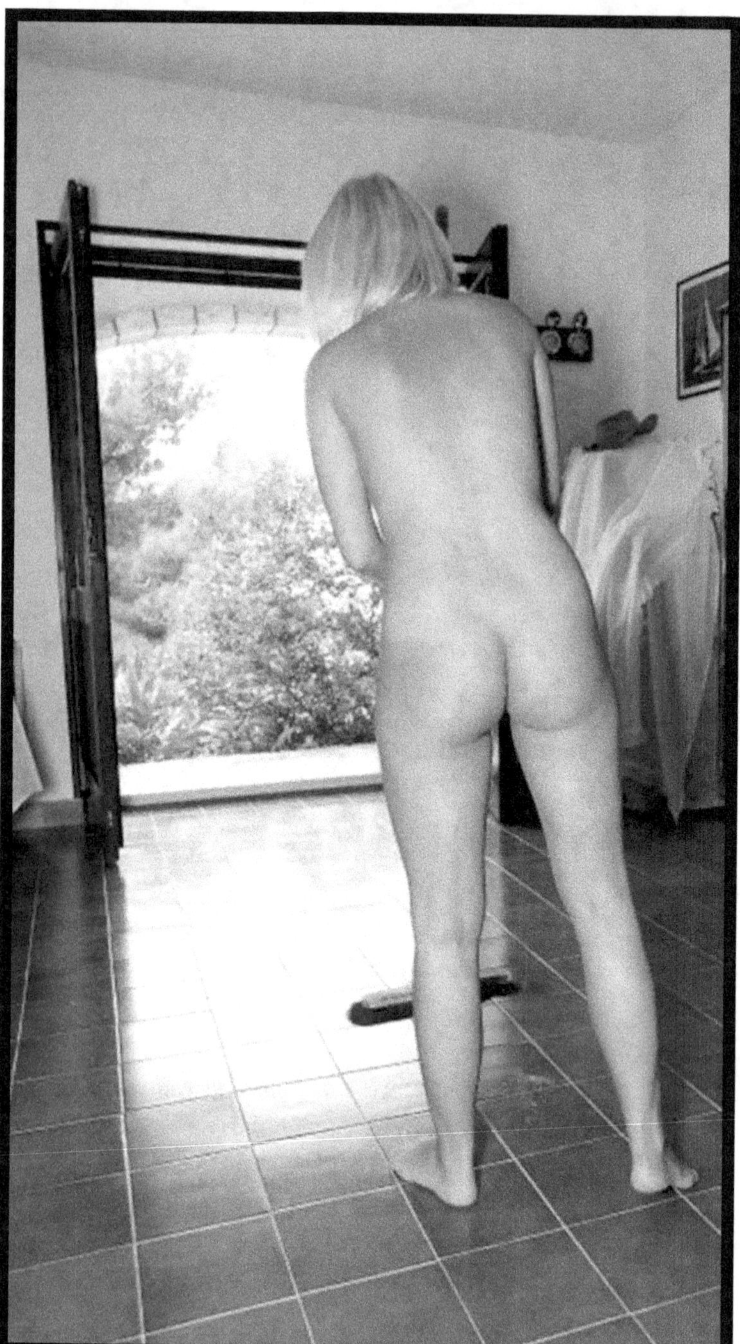

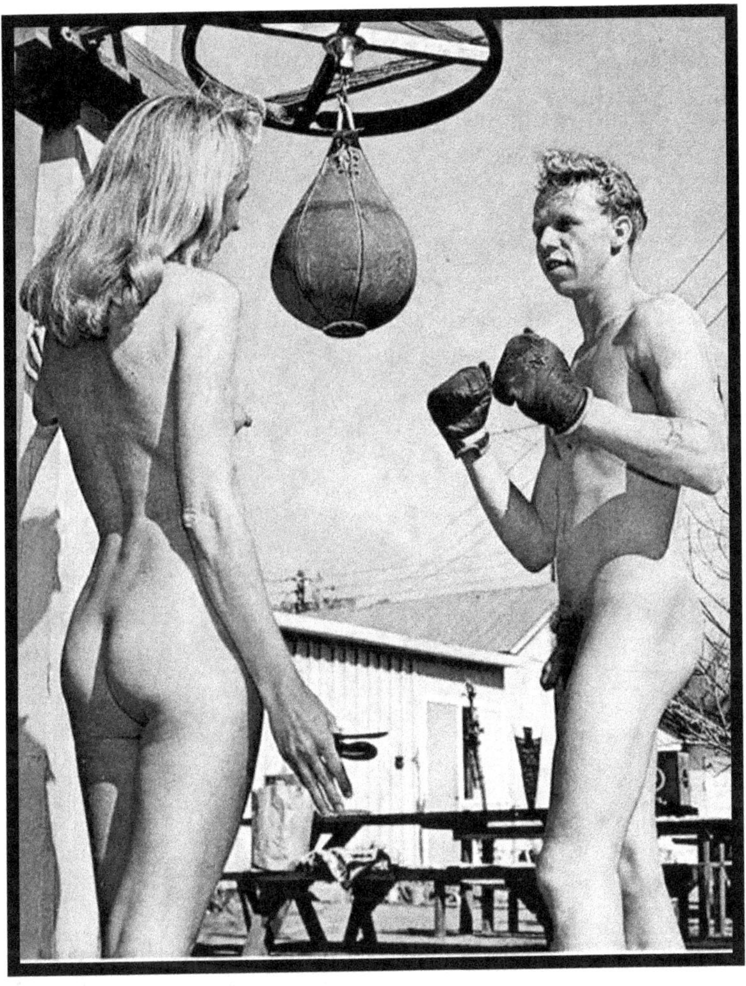

The list for nudist social events is endless, the only limit is the imagination. Always make sure to look around, especially if you're new to an area, and see what options you have.

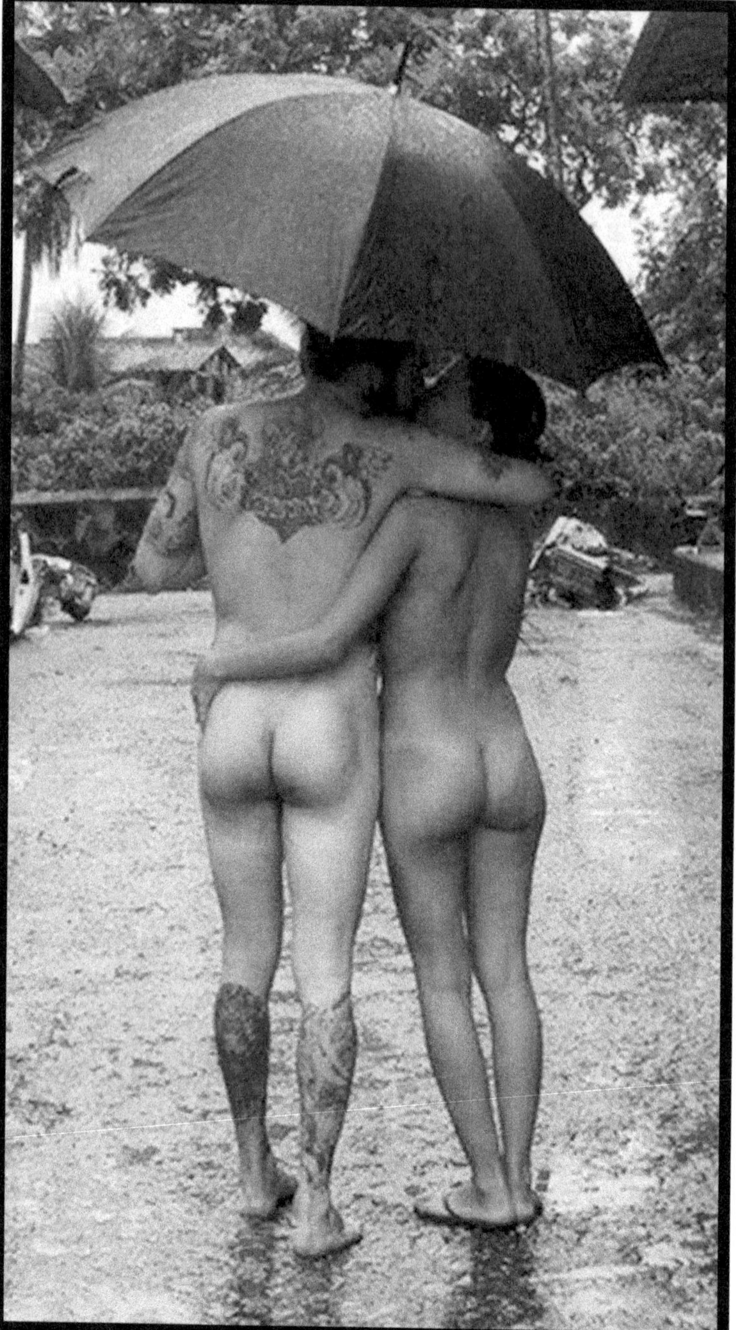

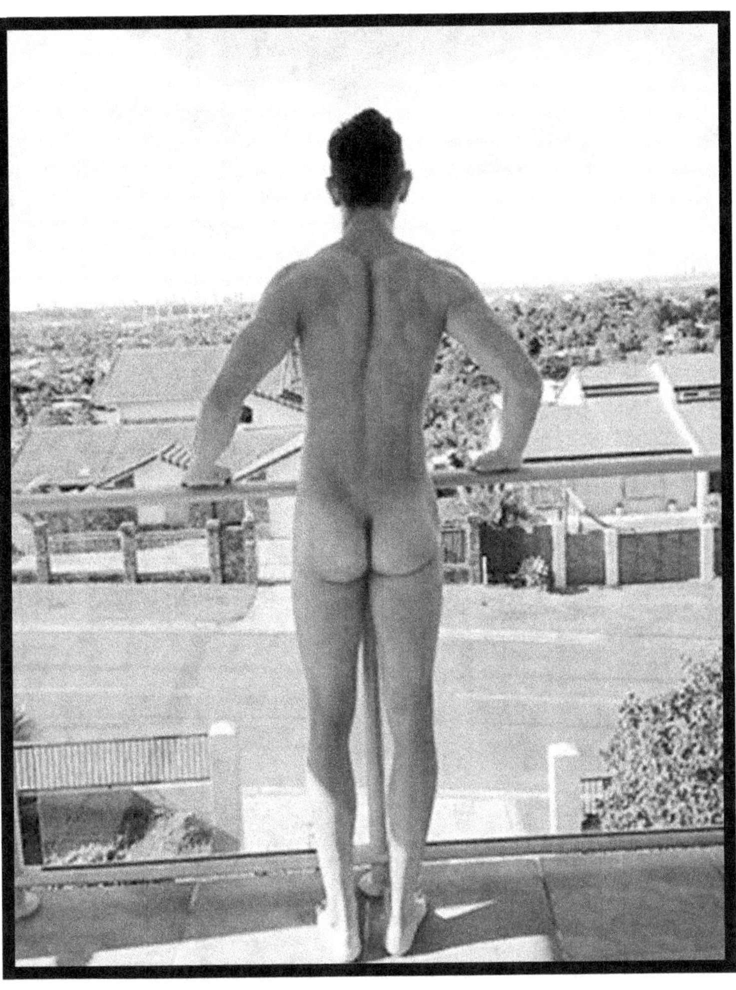

It is important however to note that some local laws restrict different types of nudity in different environments and each person should be aware of the laws and keep them in mind before organizing or attending any nudist get together. The last thing you want while you are relaxing, is to catch a legal charge.

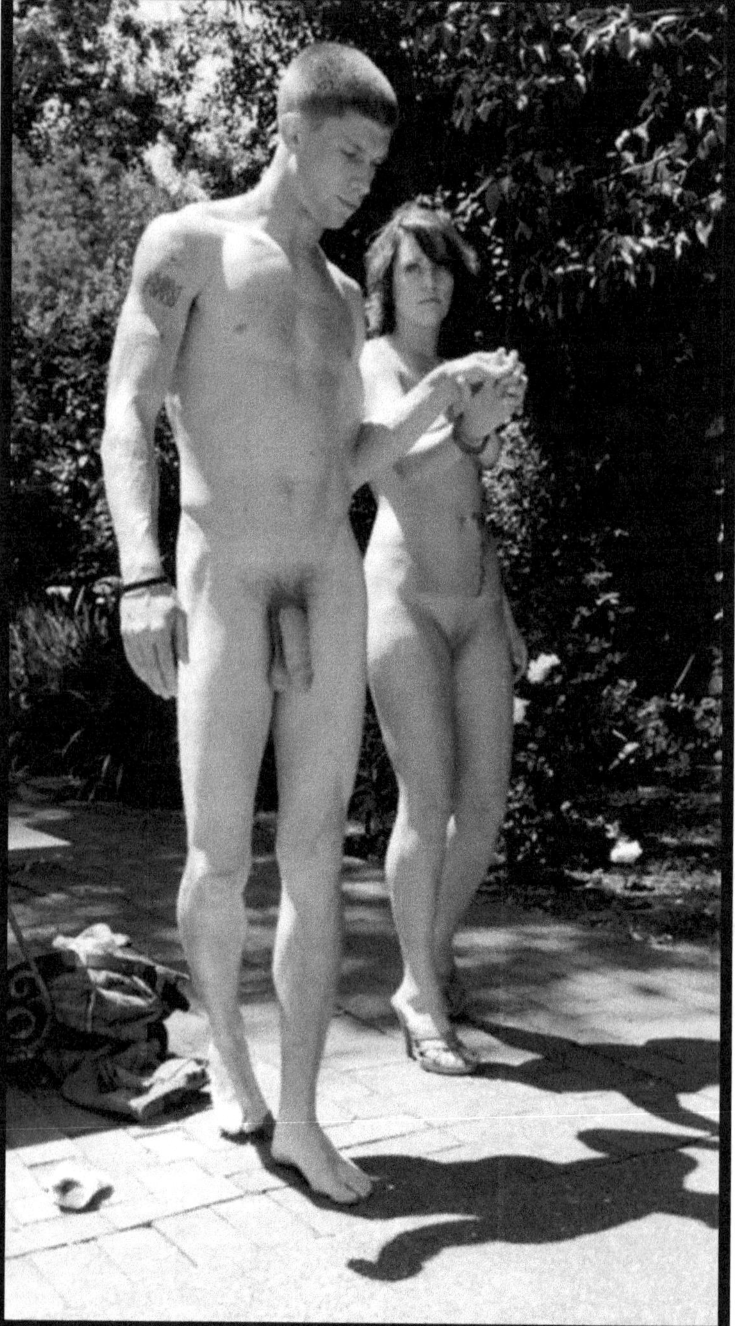

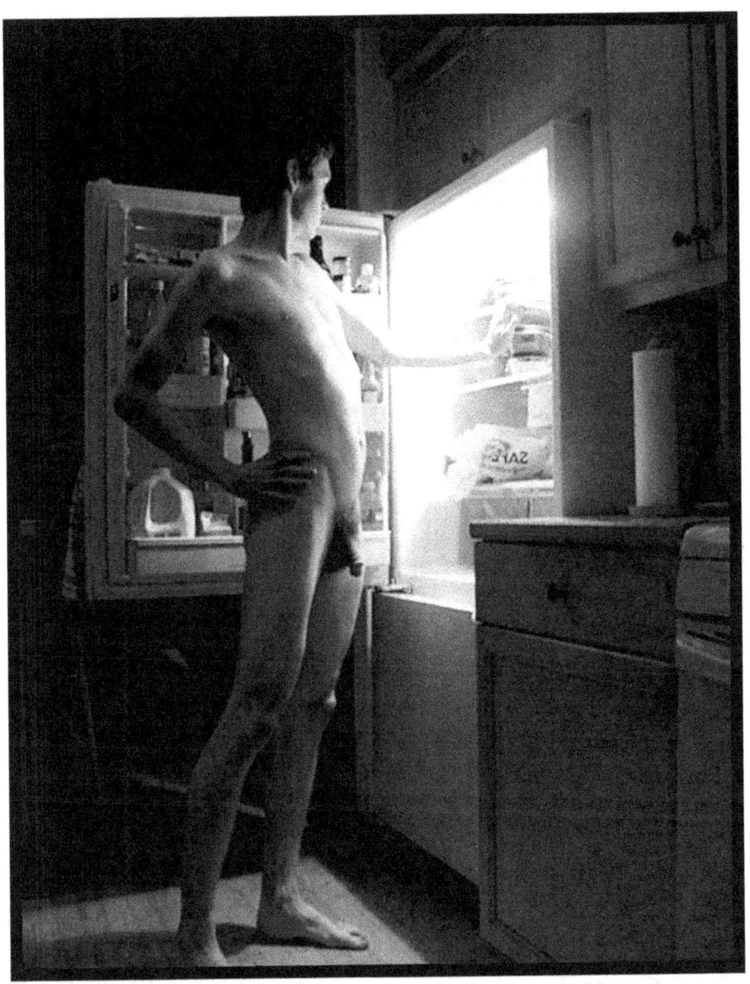

Relax and Exercise in the Nude

What more comfortable form to relax than in the nude? We've all lain in our bed nude, fresh out of the shower, refusing to get dressed, and why not? It feels so relaxing.

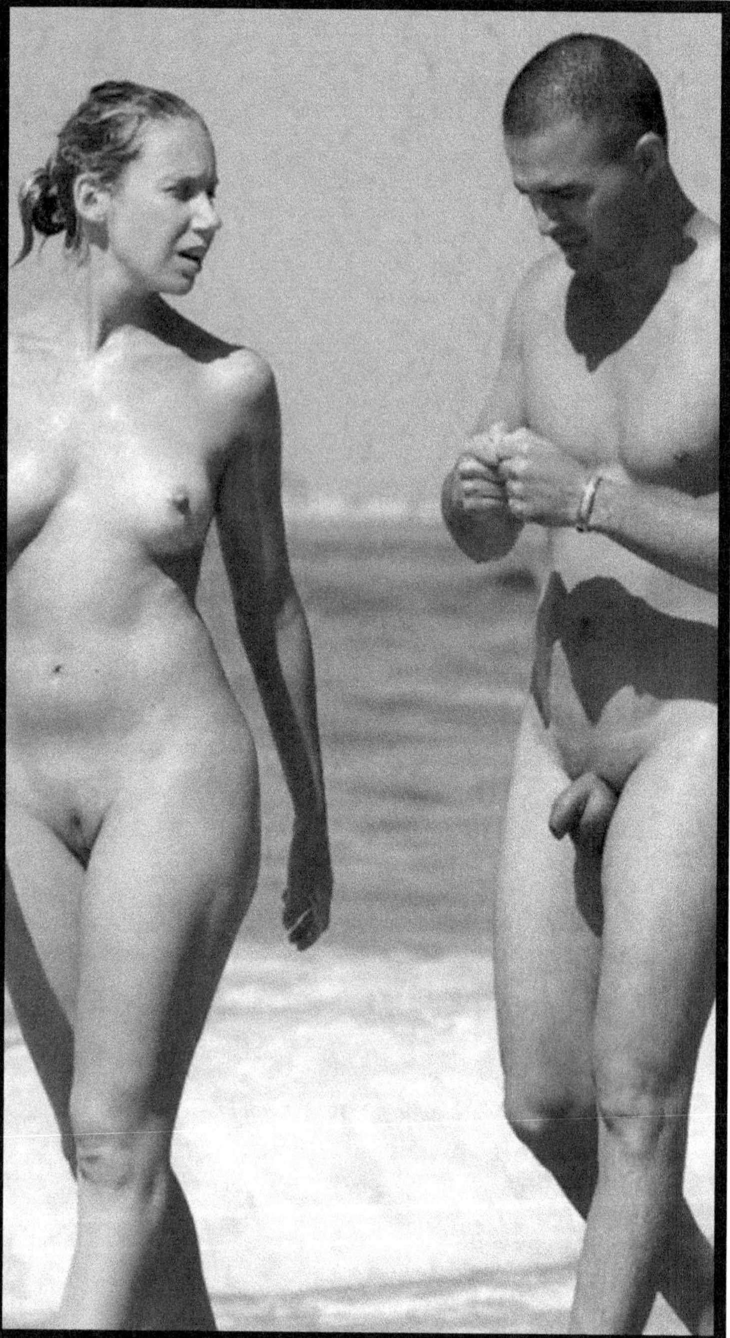

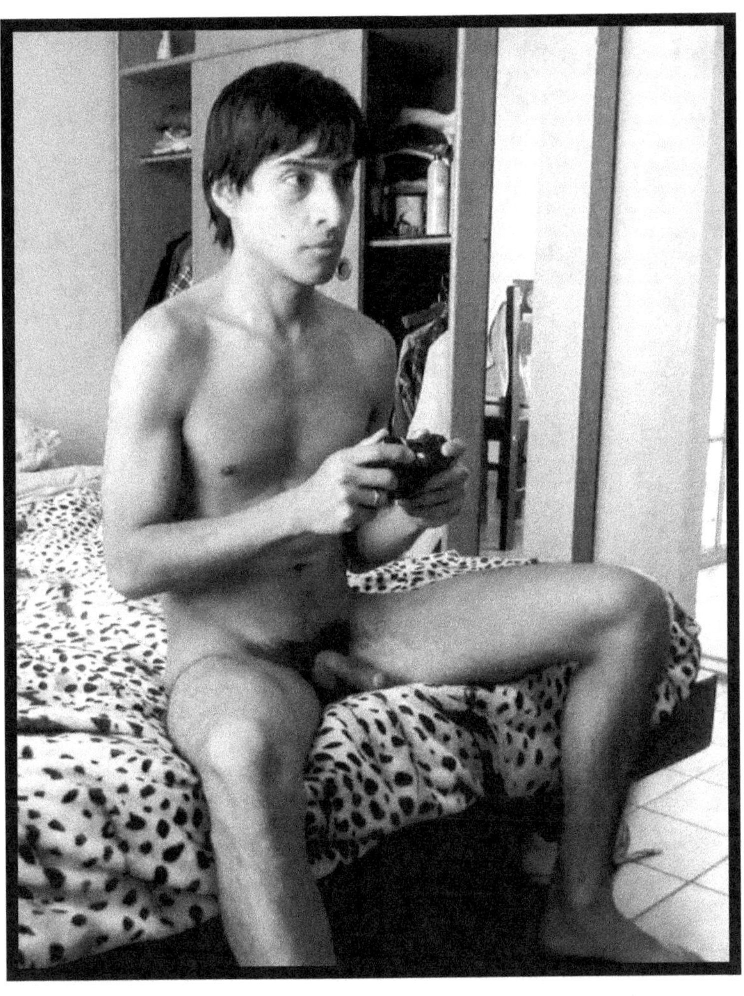

From sun bathing on a beach, to laying out in a hammock to simply spread out on the couch watching the TV and sipping a beer, what better way to relax than in your most natural form.

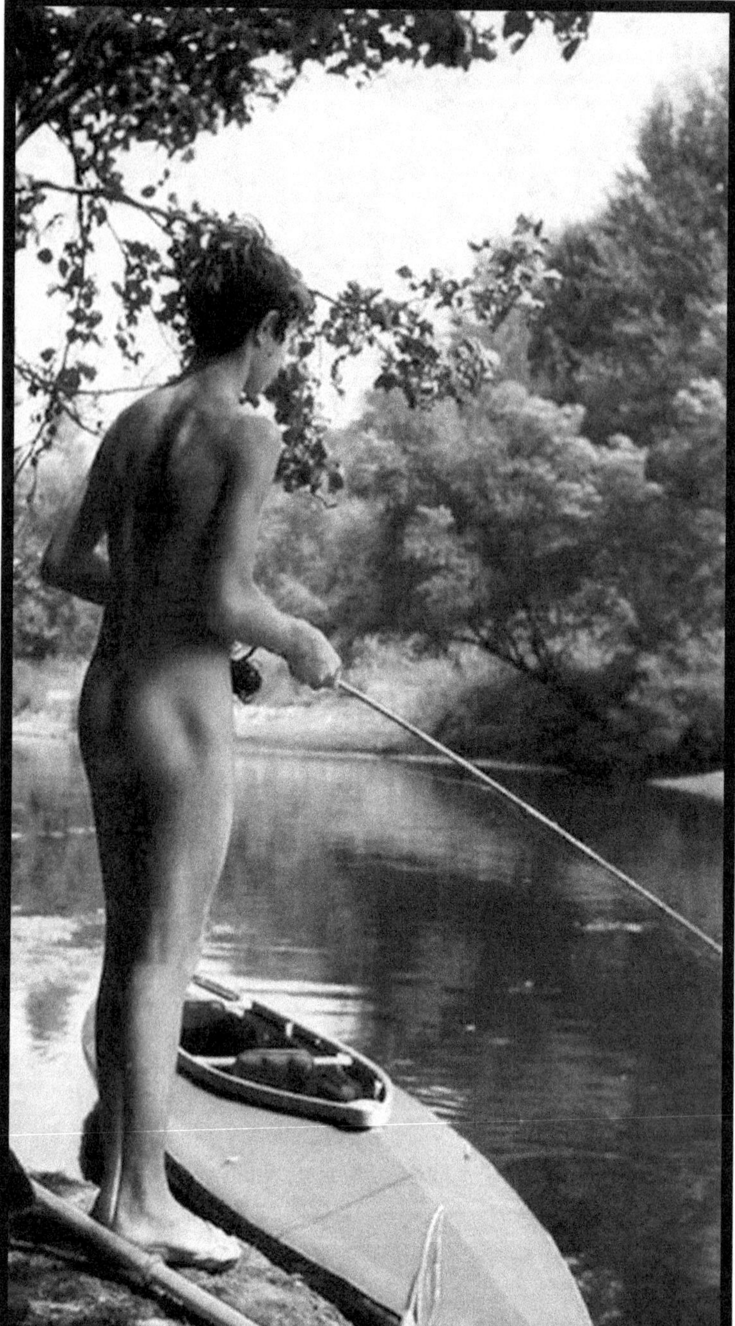

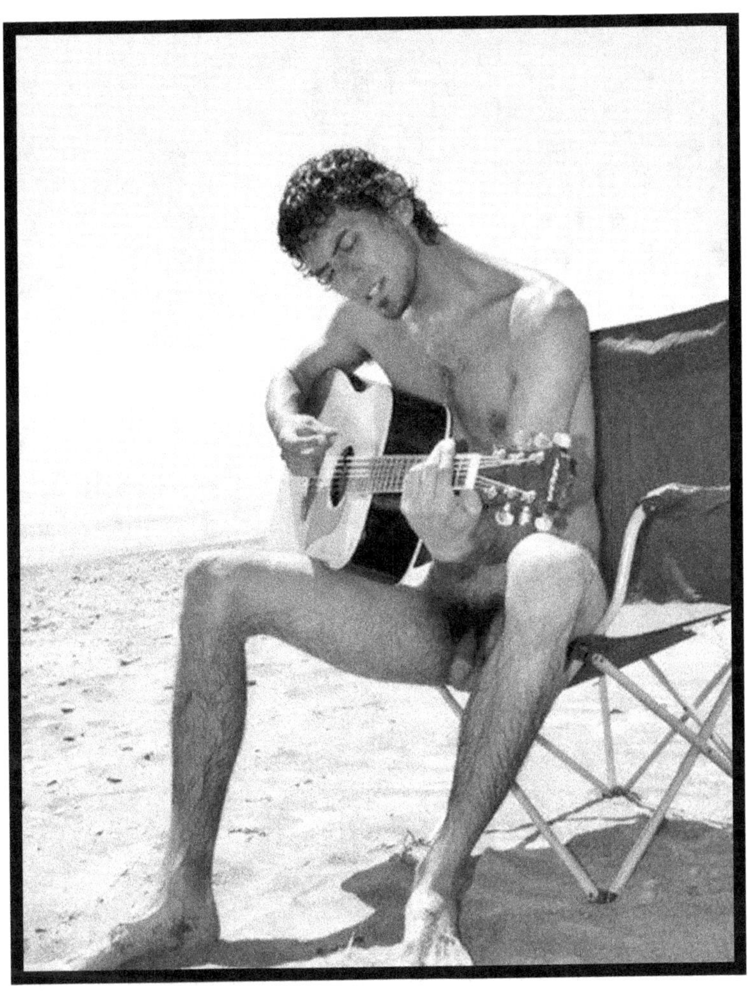

Allowing the fresh air and warm summer breeze blow against your free body can be an amazing feeling, but the relaxing qualities can also help reduce stress and help you enjoy life more.

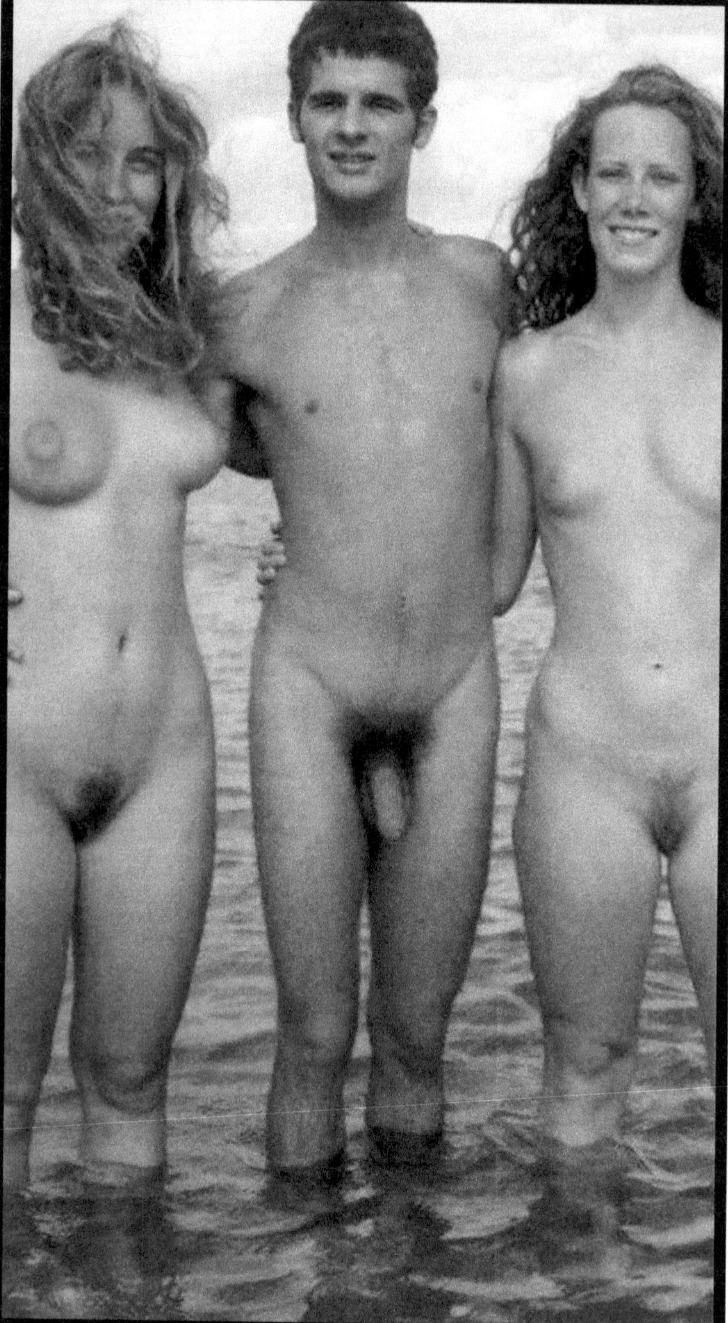

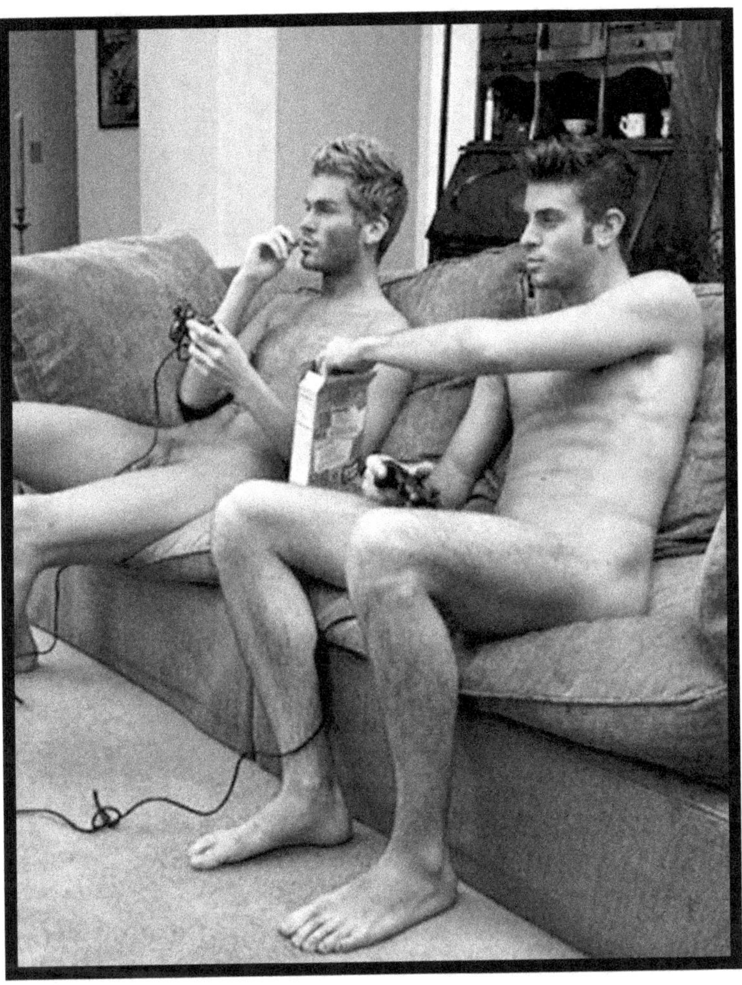

There have been several occasions where I have had friends over and we just sat around nude and played on my Xbox or watched movies. In fact, I had a best friend growing up, that whenever we would hang out at his house, and his parents weren't home, we'd literally spend the whole day lying around his house nude.

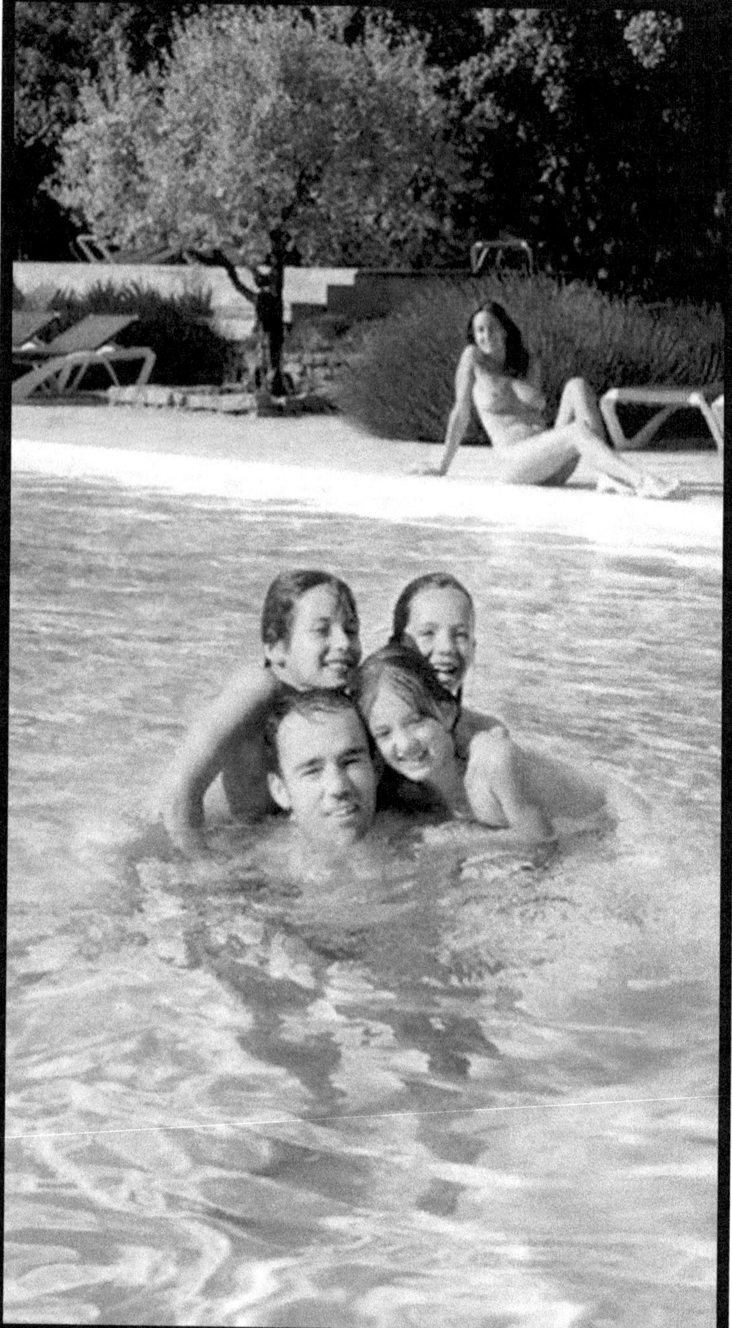

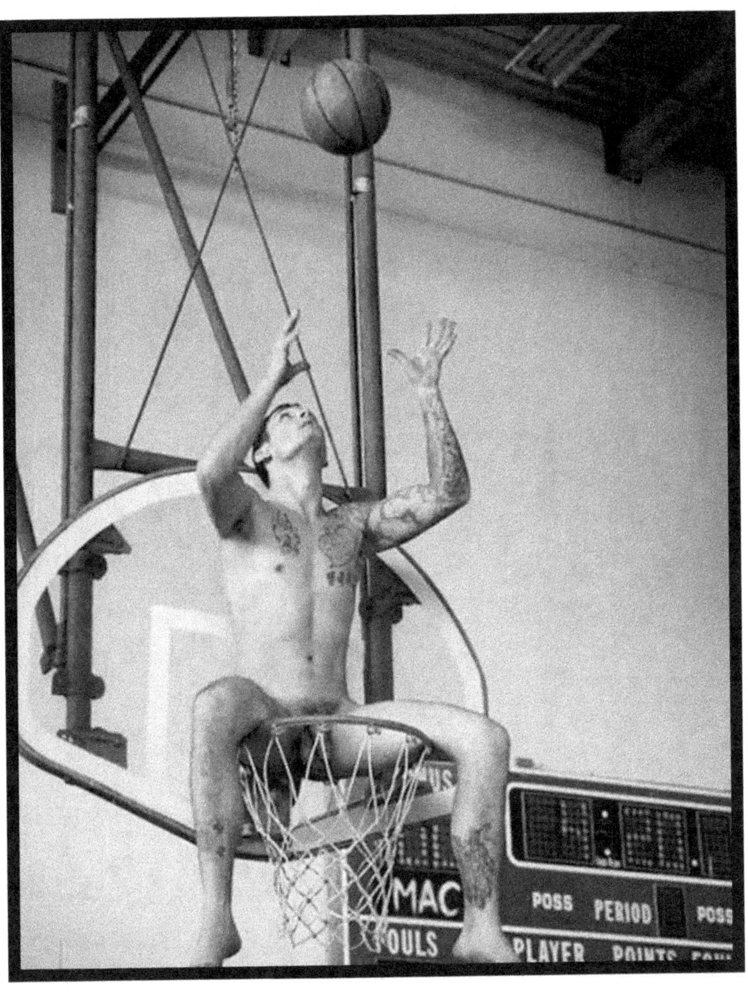

Exercising nude is amazing for your body, medically, as well as just being more enjoyable.

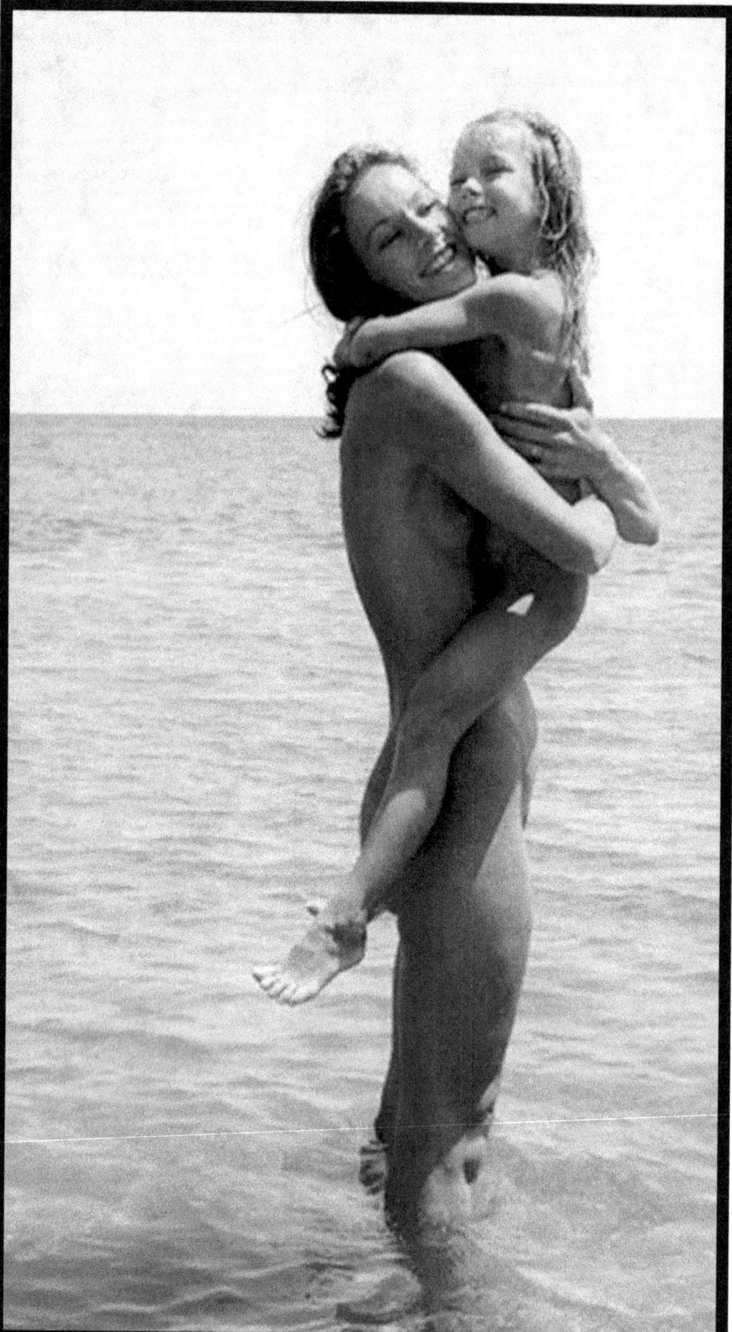

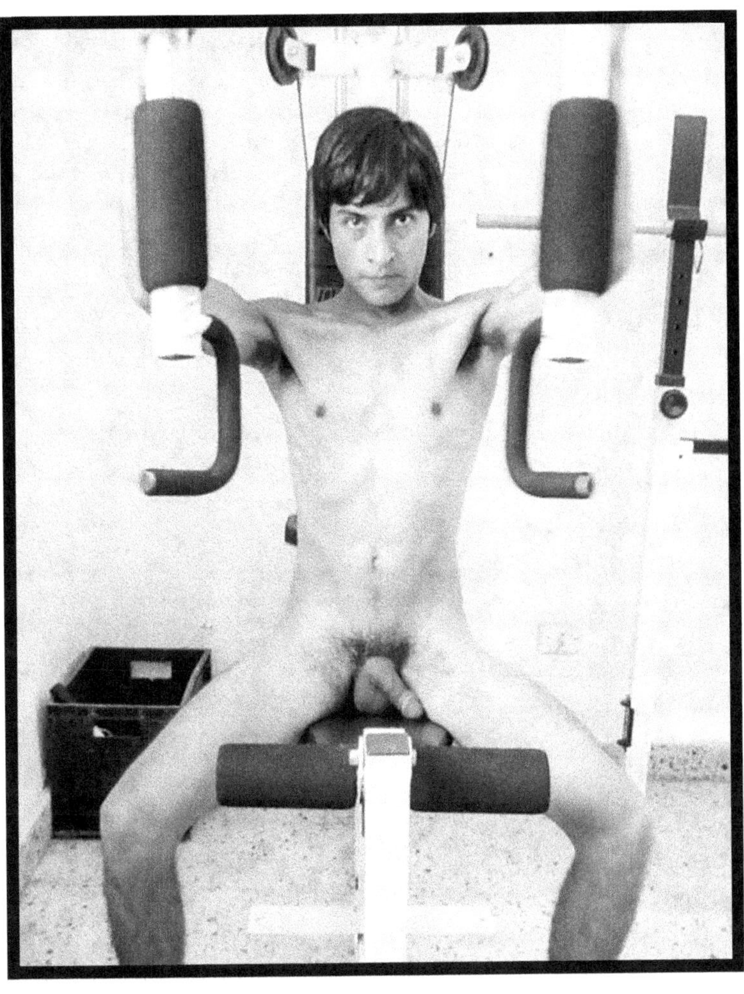

If you have a home gym, or a gym that allows such, working out nude is great way to free yourself. Allowing your body's natural full range of motion, unrestricted by clothing, and allowing your body to sweat and cool itself naturally, is the healthiest way of working out.

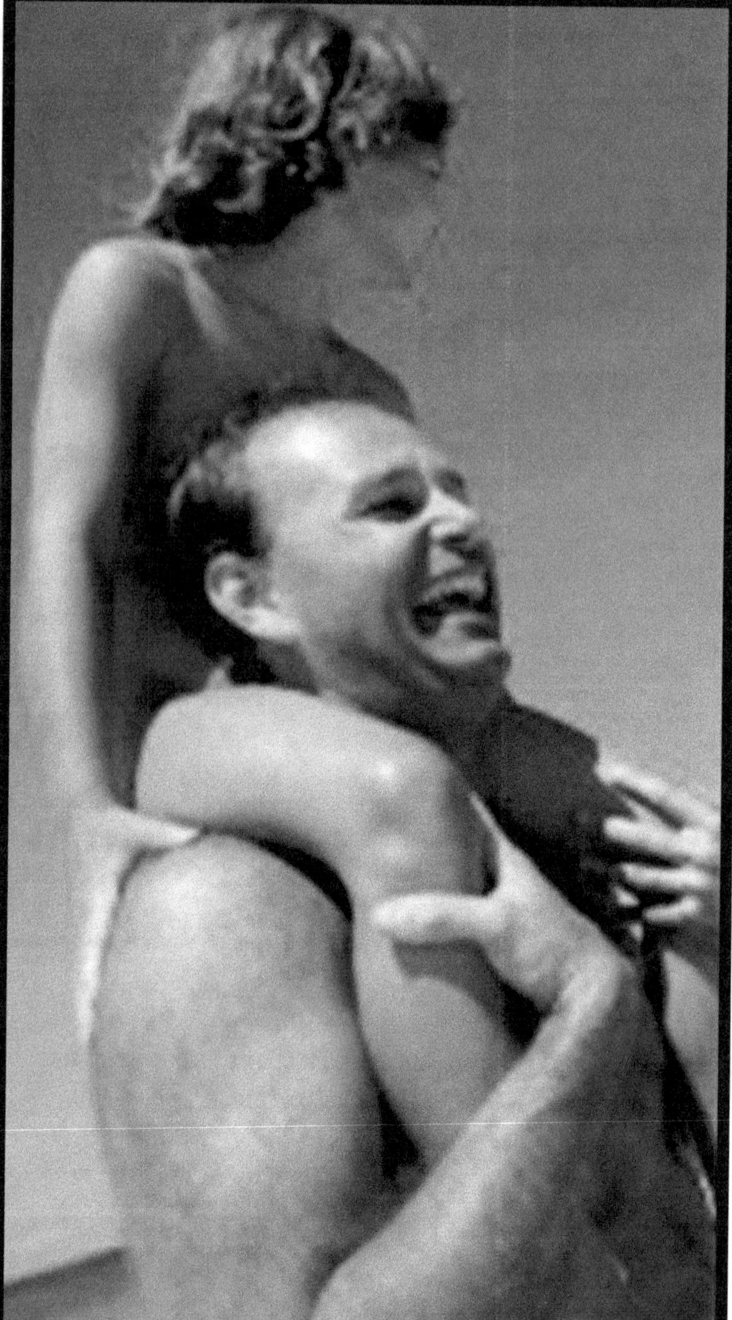

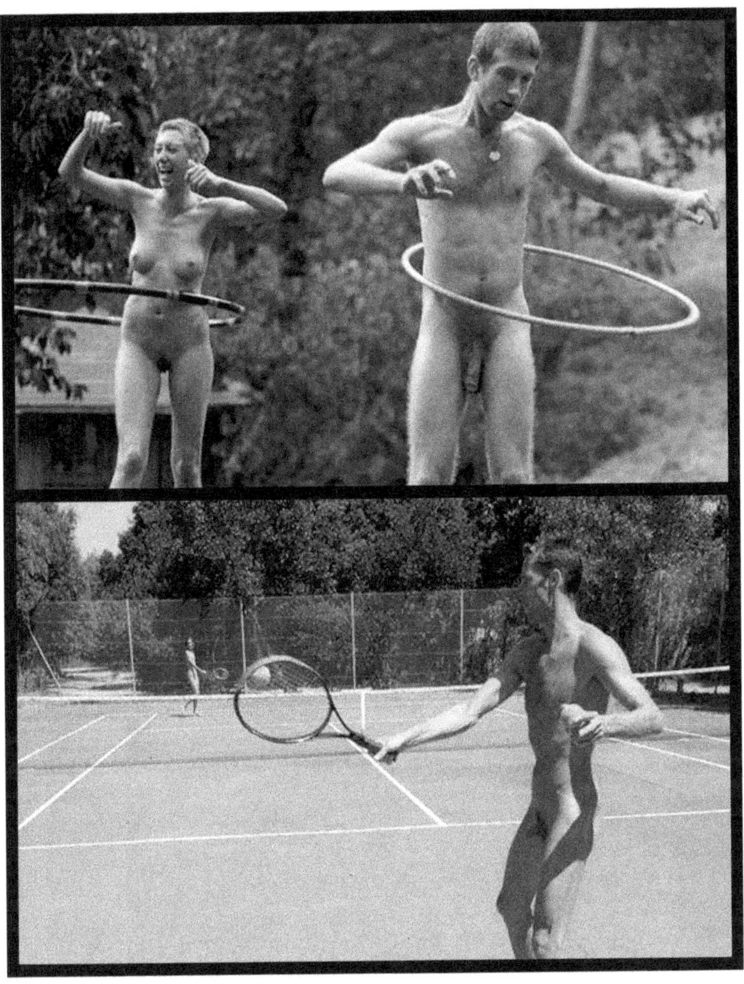

Allowing your naked body to breathe during exercising will keep
your body temperature down, preventing you from
overheating.
Conversely, wearing clothing while exercising will trap the sweat
against your body, preventing the toxins that are contained in
sweat, to leave your body. Also, trapping sweat against your
body can cause chaffing, due to the salt build up, caused by
body sweat.

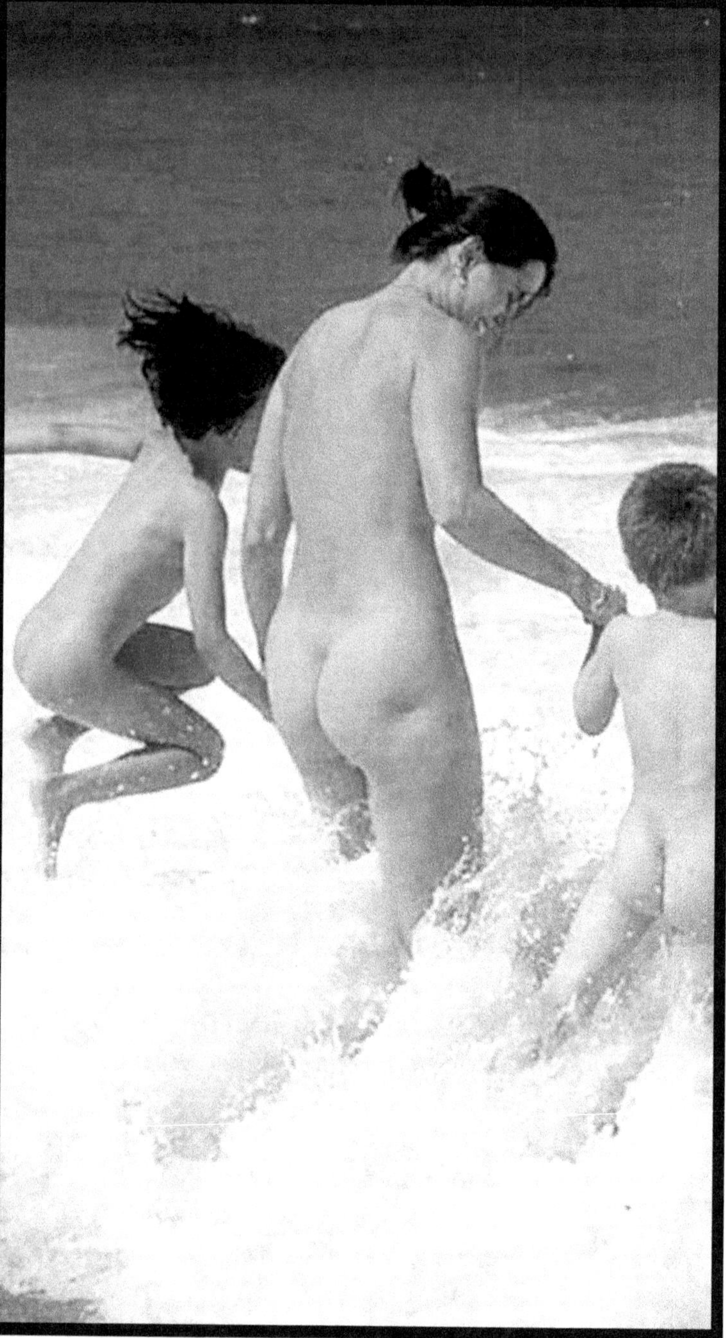

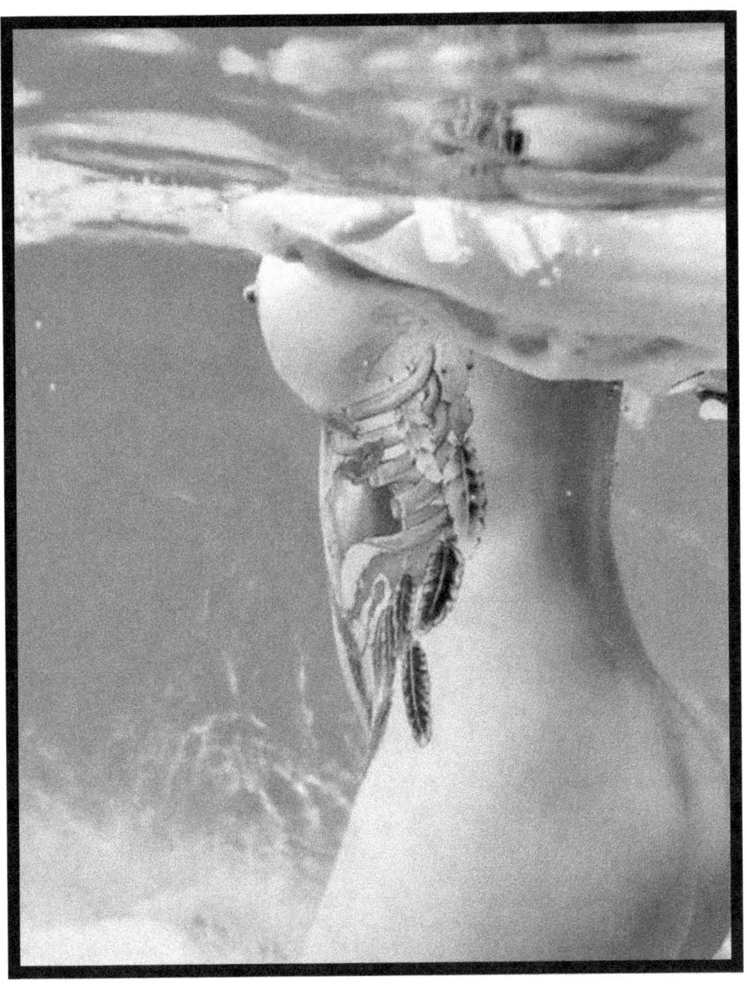

Another great note, not only is exercising great for your health, it is also a great life hack, and you no longer have to wash sweaty gym clothes.

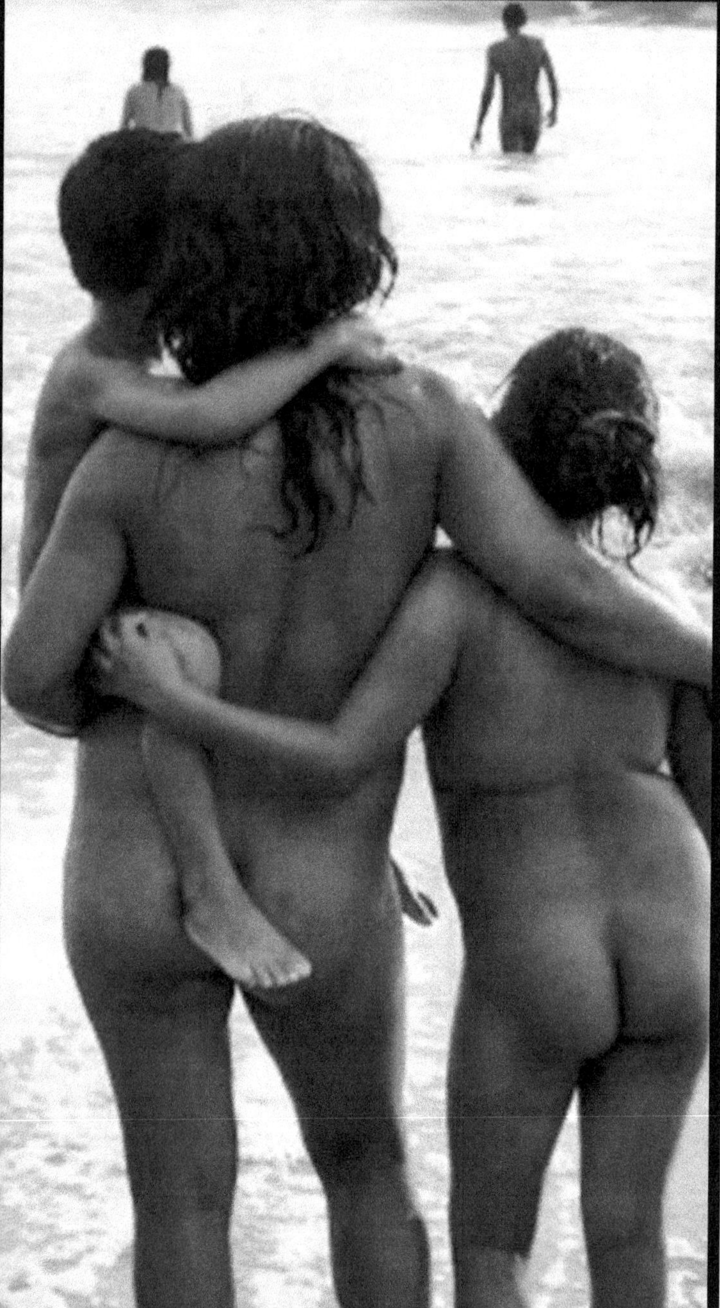

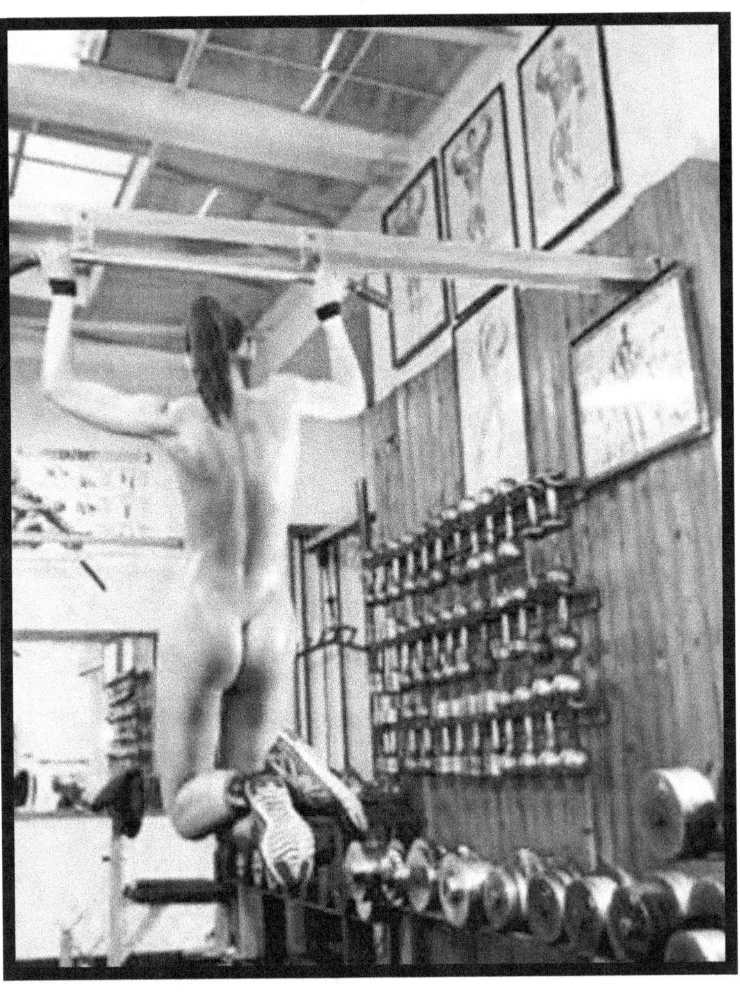

Obviously you need to make sure that whenever you are sweating that you are doing everything you need to maintain a sanitary environment, putting down a towel when you sit down and wiping down equipment and workout surfaces whenever necessary.

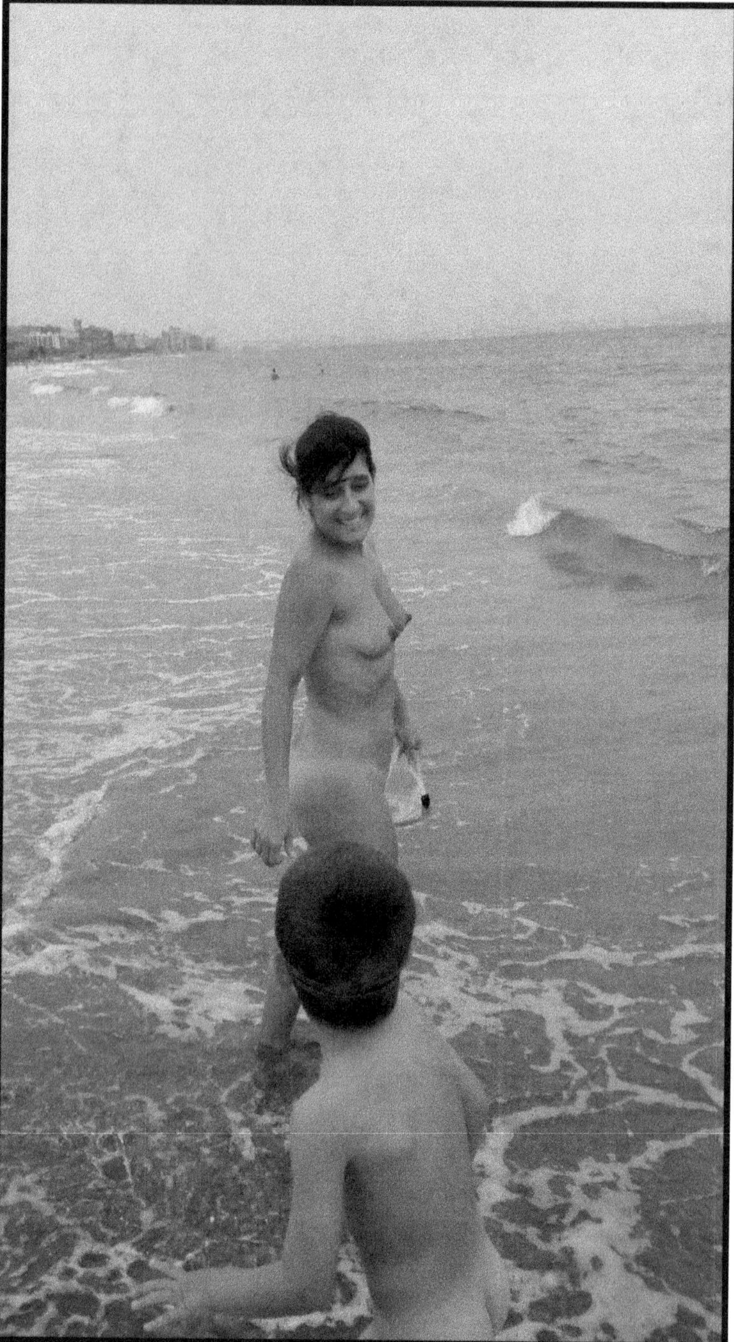

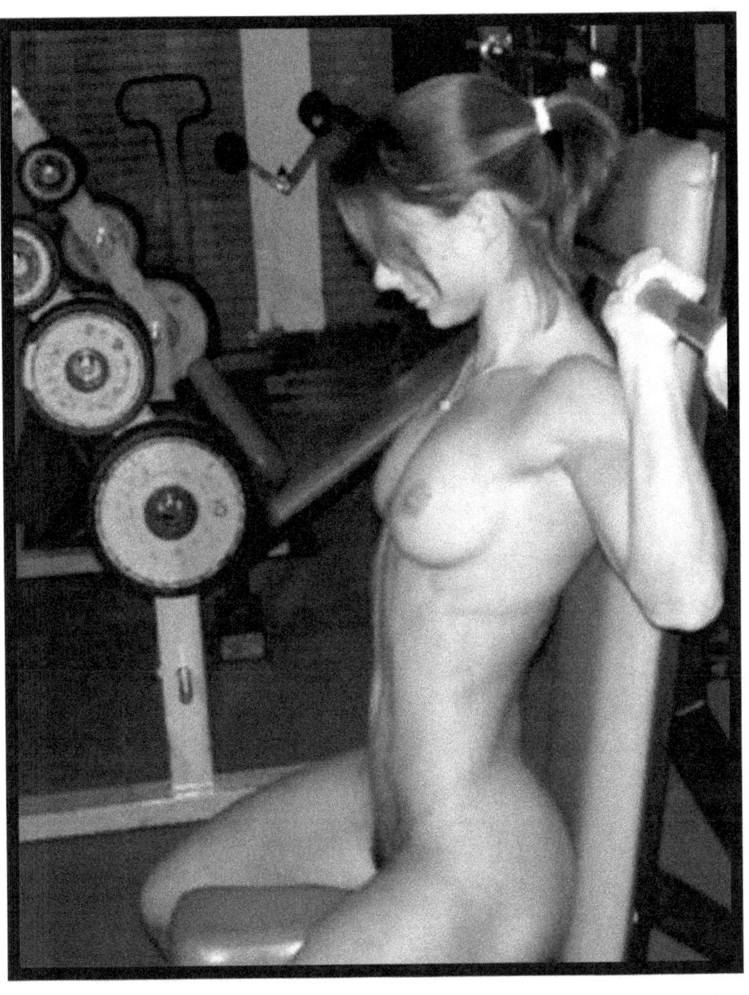

It is also customary in most nudist environments to ask friends and guests to sit on a towel, in order to maintain sanitation levels. Do not be offended if you are asked to do so, in fact, I recommend that you always bring a towel when you do anything nude, just in case.

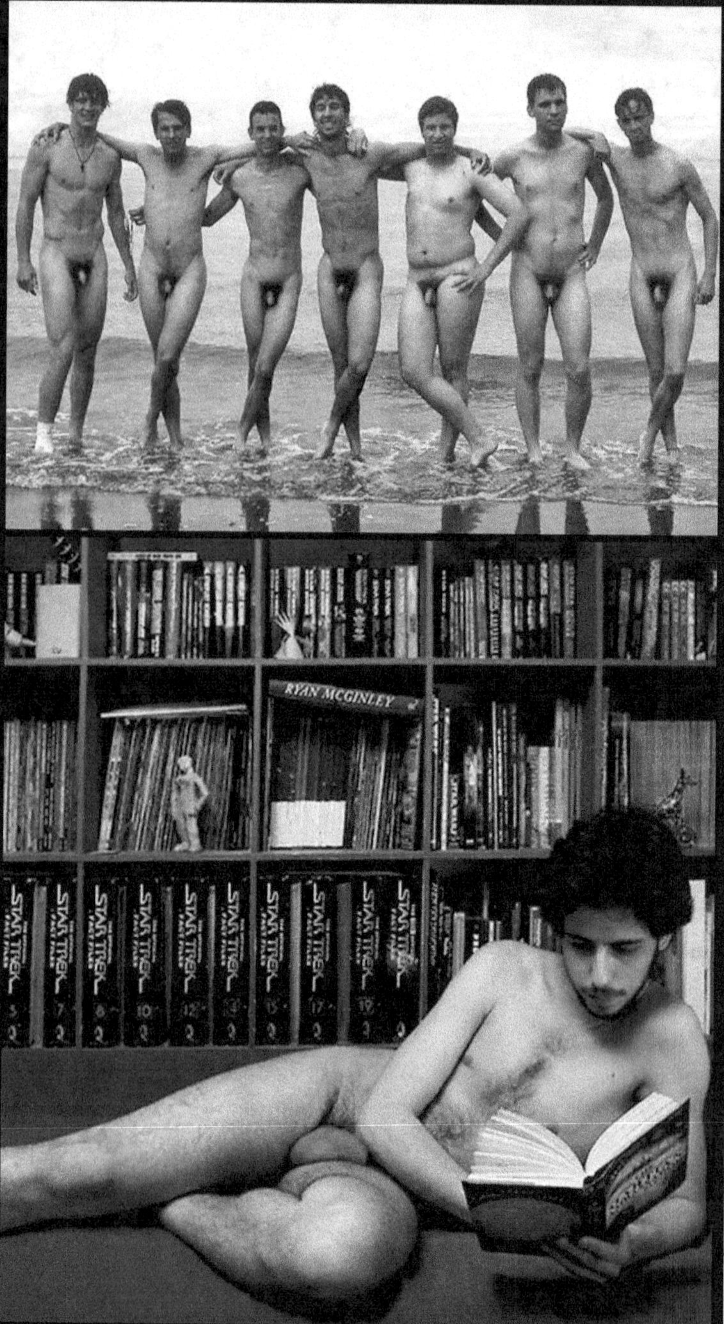

RYAN MCGINLEY
STAR TREK

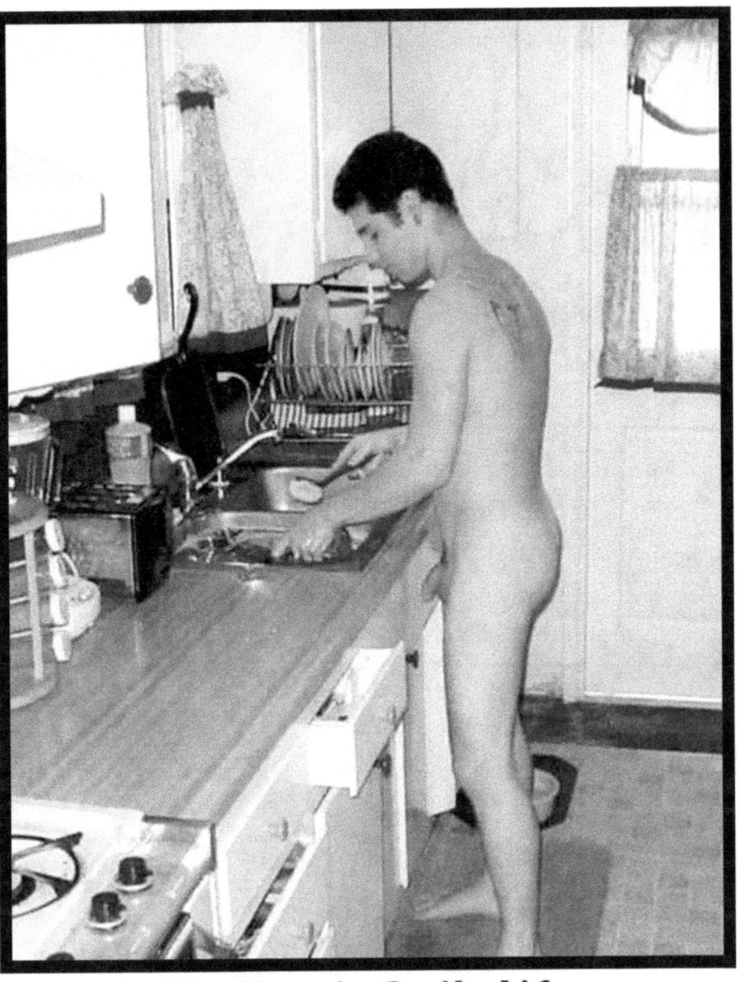

Nudism in Daily Life

Nudism is daily life is the same as anyone else with a few exceptions. While you will need to put on clothes before you can leave your house, what you do at home is the same as anyone else, just free of the restrictions of clothing.

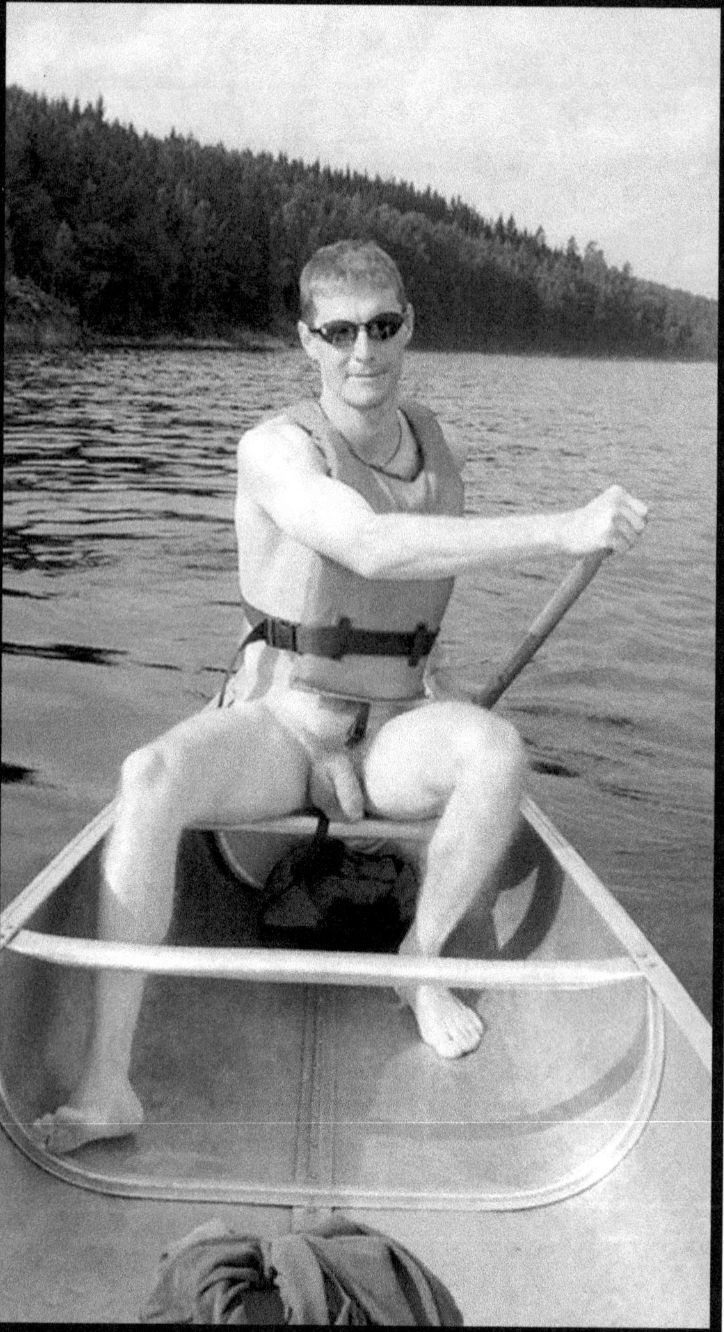

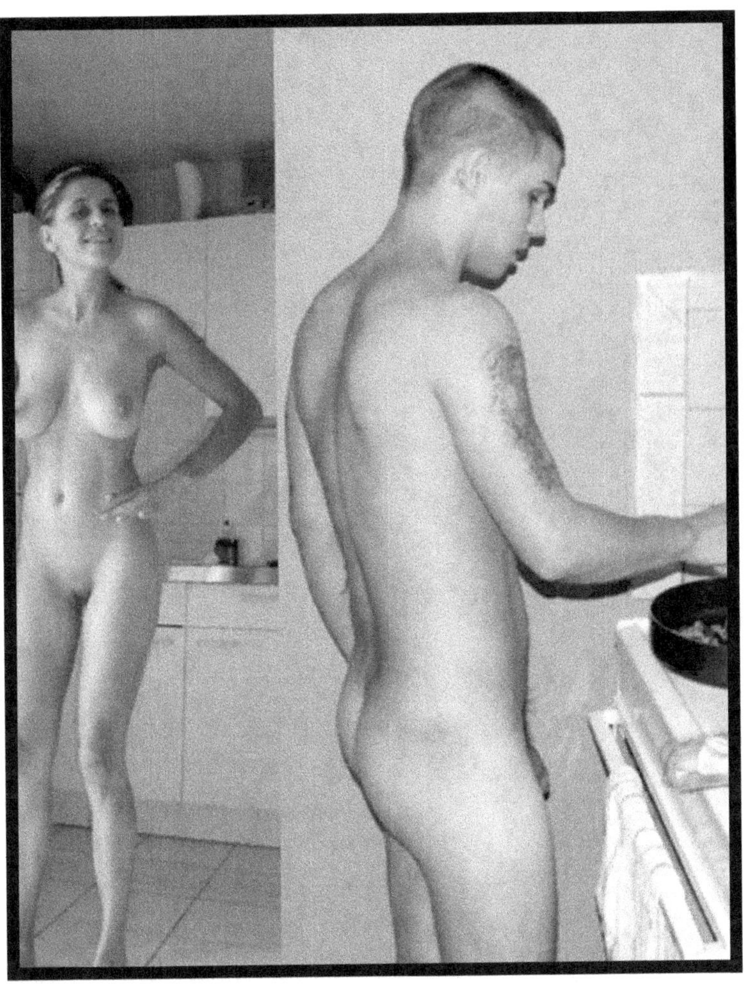

Cooking nude is an interesting experience, but should be done with a fair bit of caution. Simply throwing something in the microwave, toasting some bread in a toaster, or even cooking some eggs on the stove is no big deal.

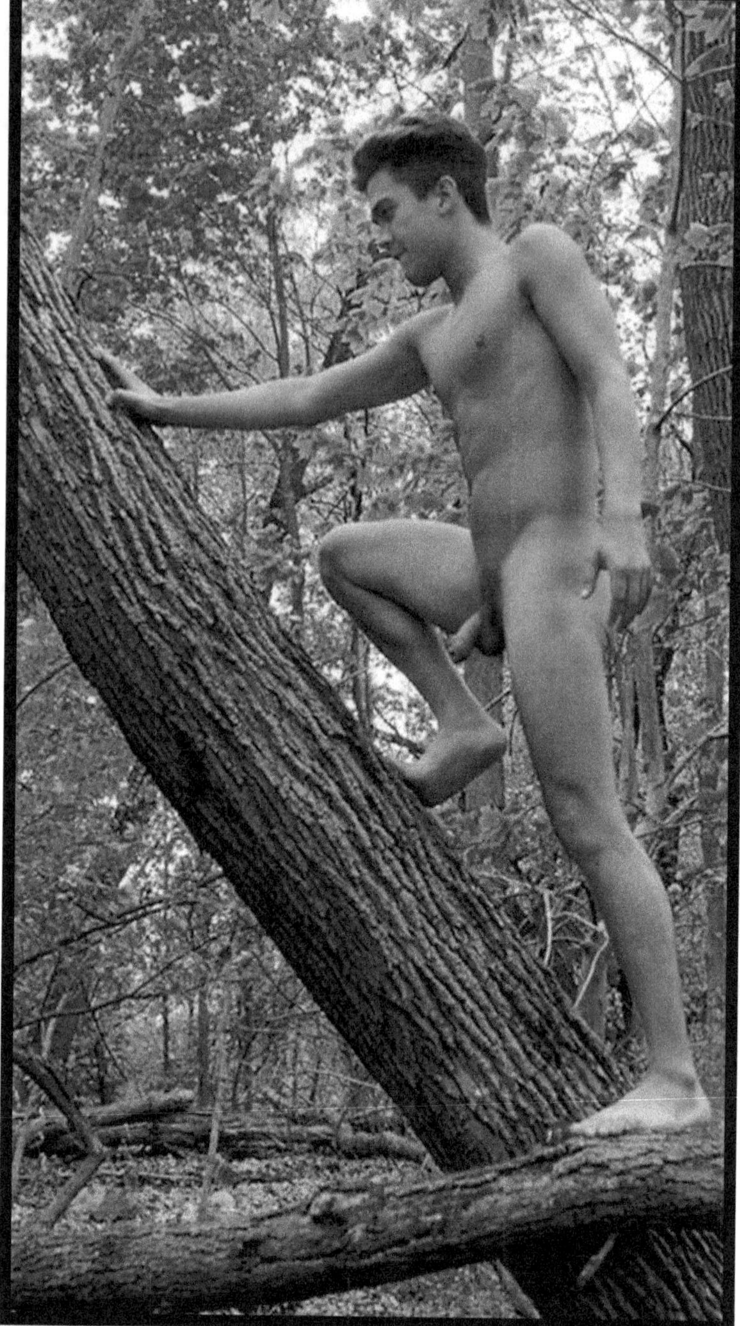

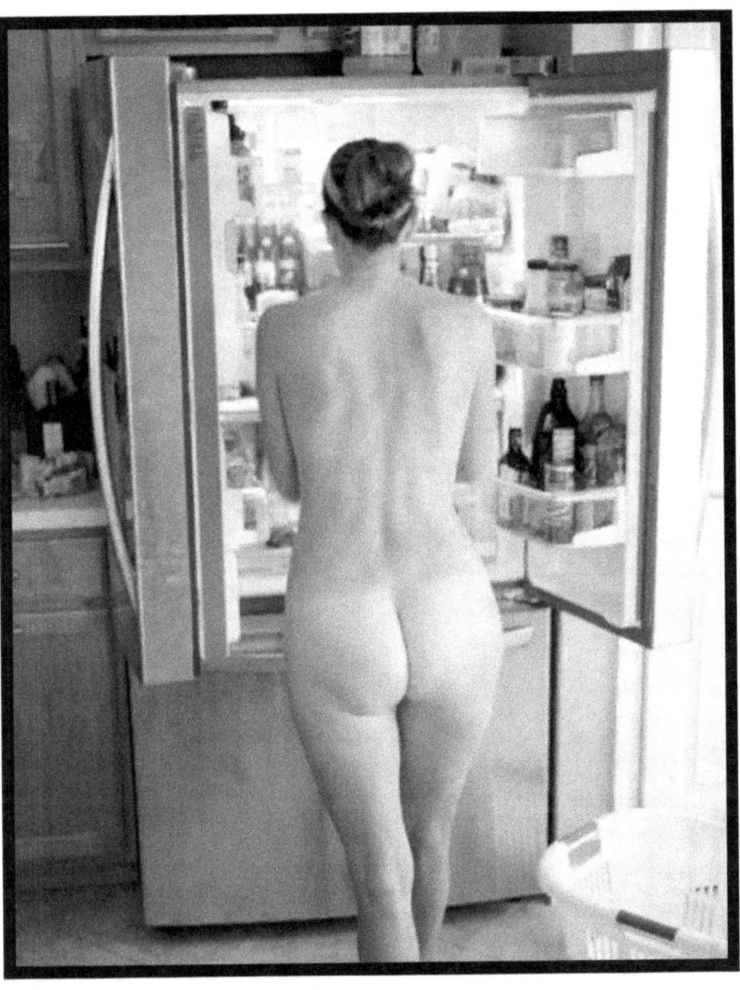

But you should be cautious when it comes to making some bacon for your eggs, or frying some vegetables in a skillet, as without clothing you have nothing to protect your bare skin from flying grease.

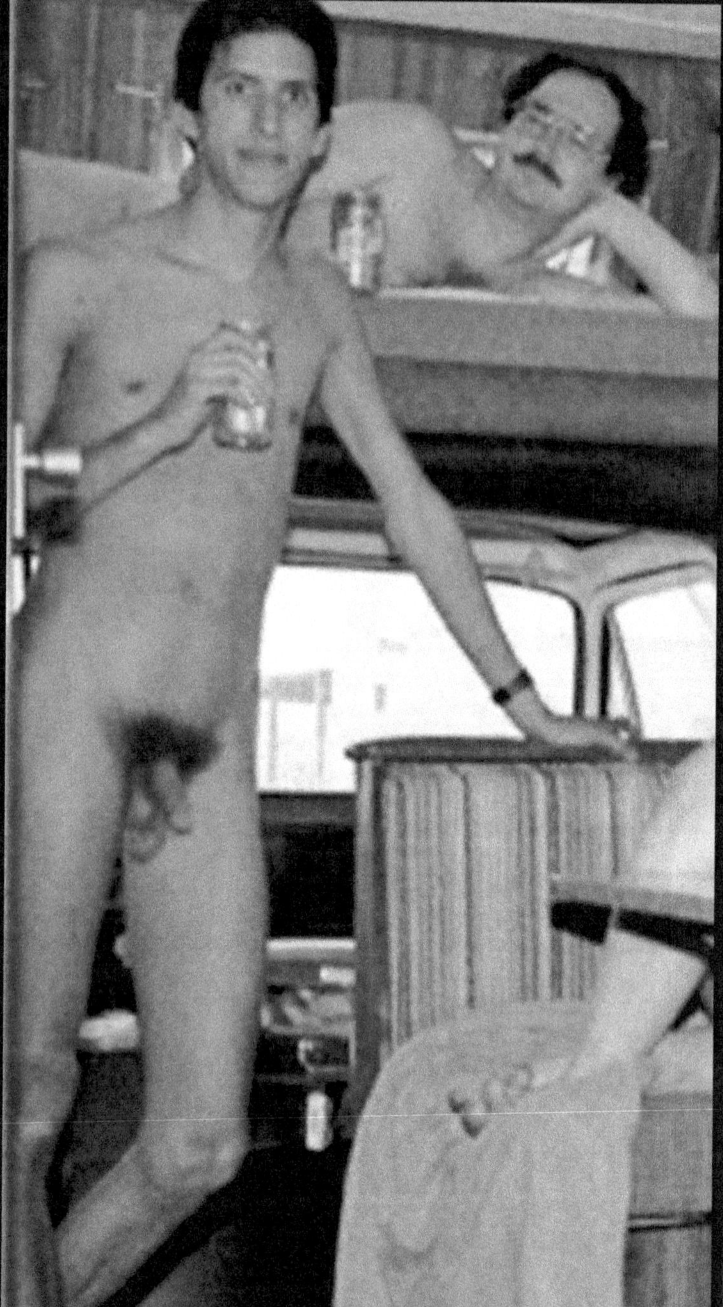

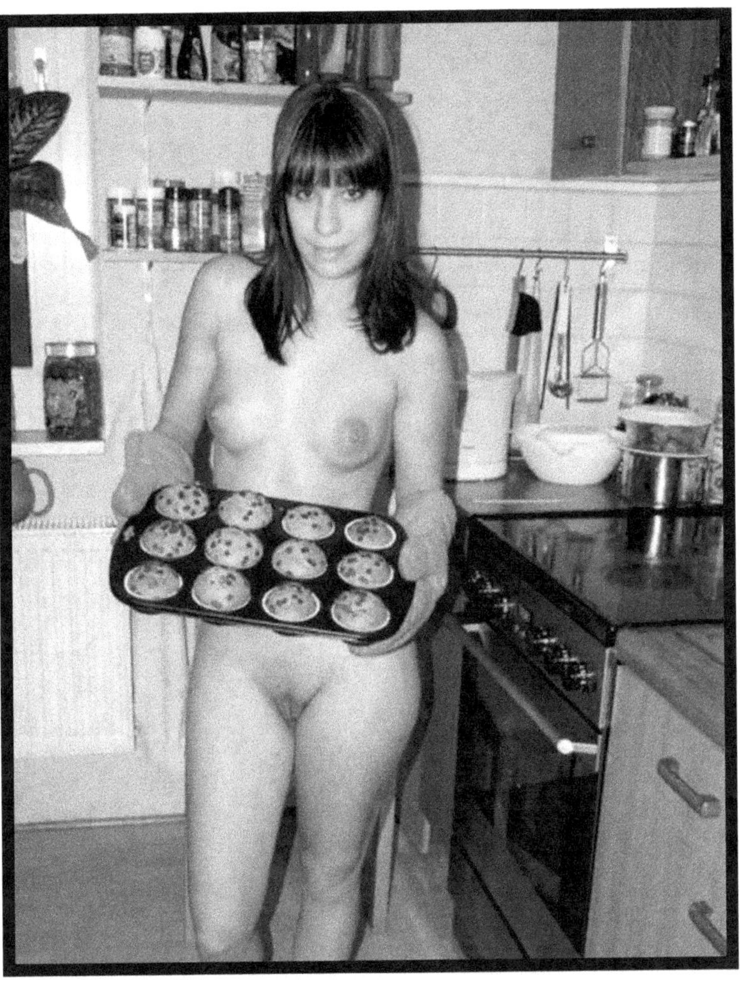

I personally enjoy cooking and baking nude, especially when baking, the kitchen can get pretty hot, so being nude is more favorable anyway. One recommendation, when cooking and similarly with cleaning with harsh chemicals, where an apron.

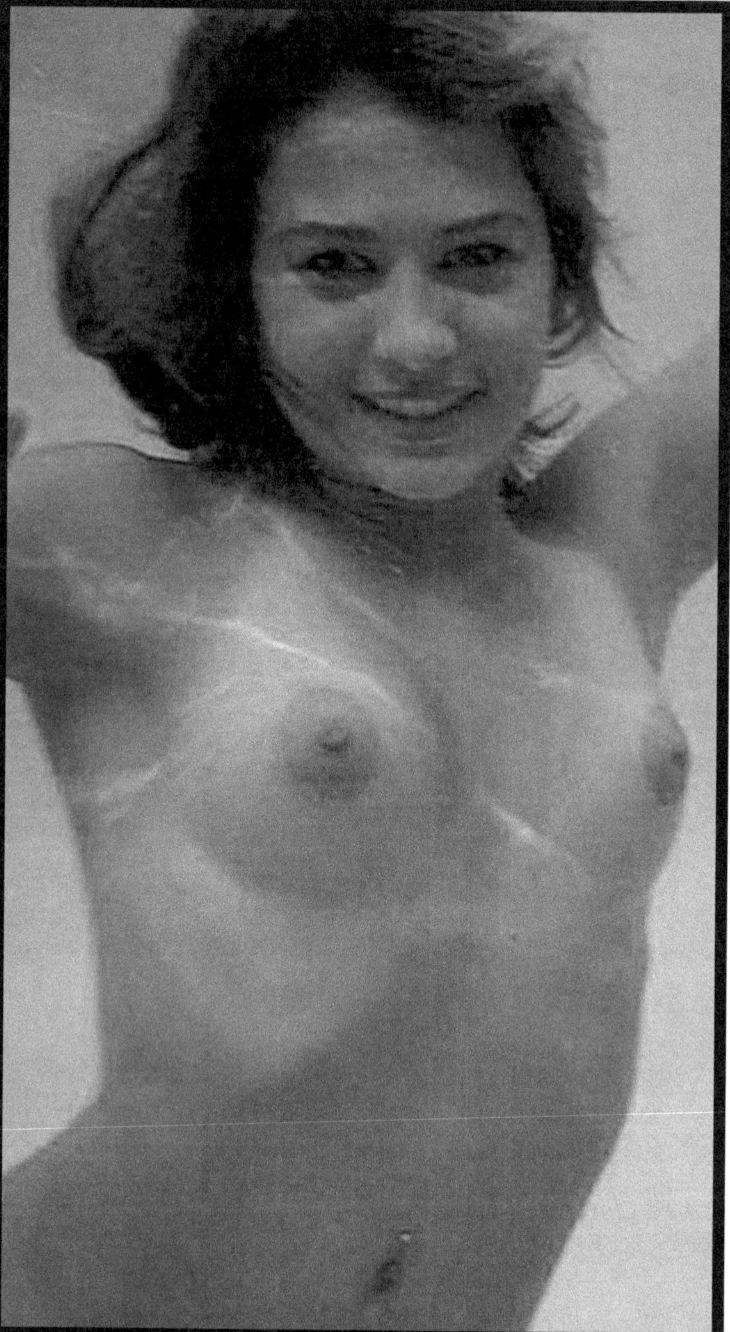

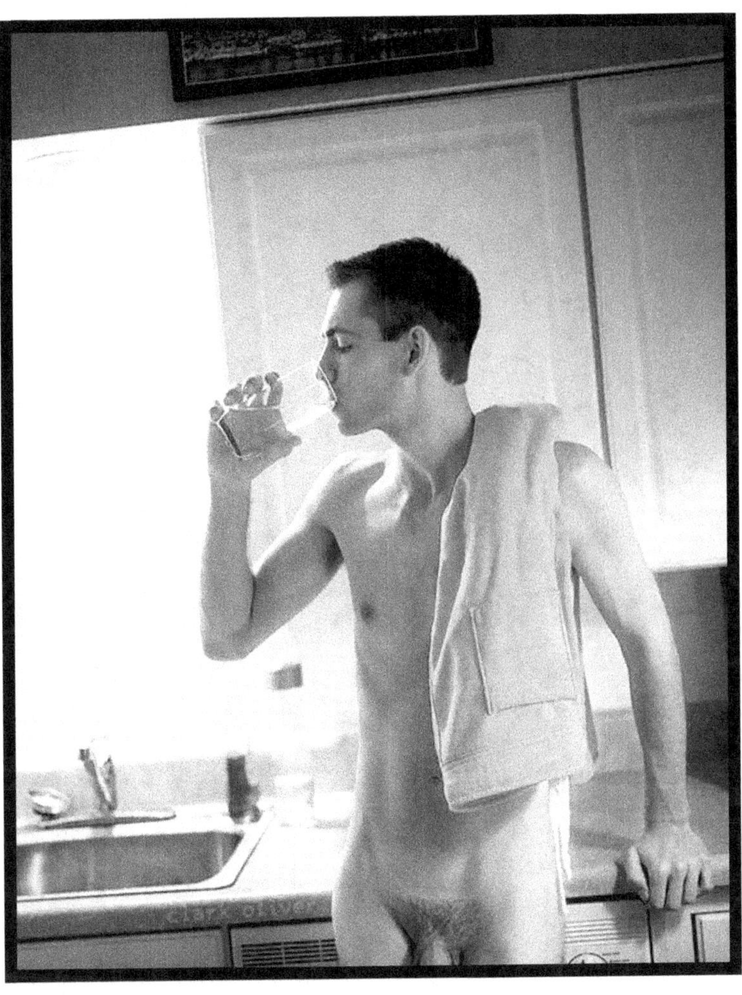

Dusting and vacuuming nude aren't the forms of cleaning that are possible to do nude. Most of your everyday chemicals, like Windex and Lysol, are perfectly safe to work around nude. I would be more careful with things such as Tilex or other harsher chemicals that use bleach.

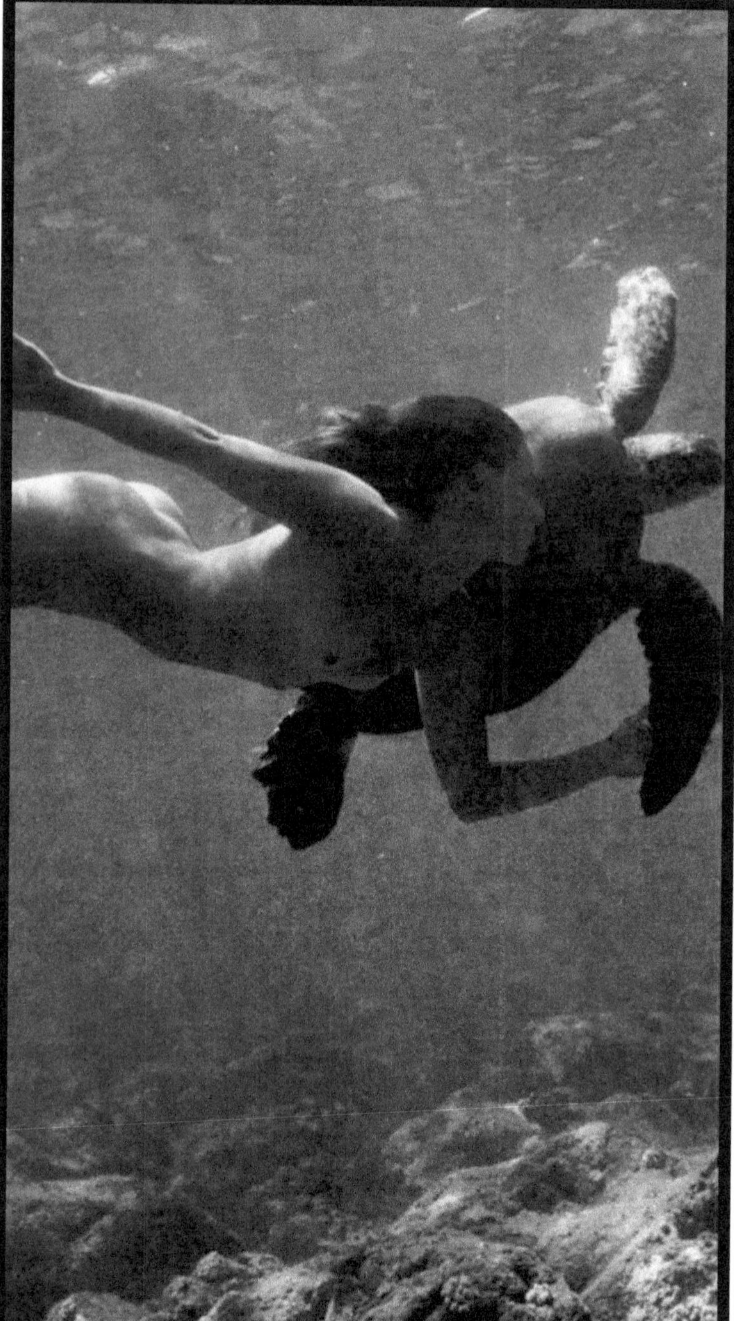

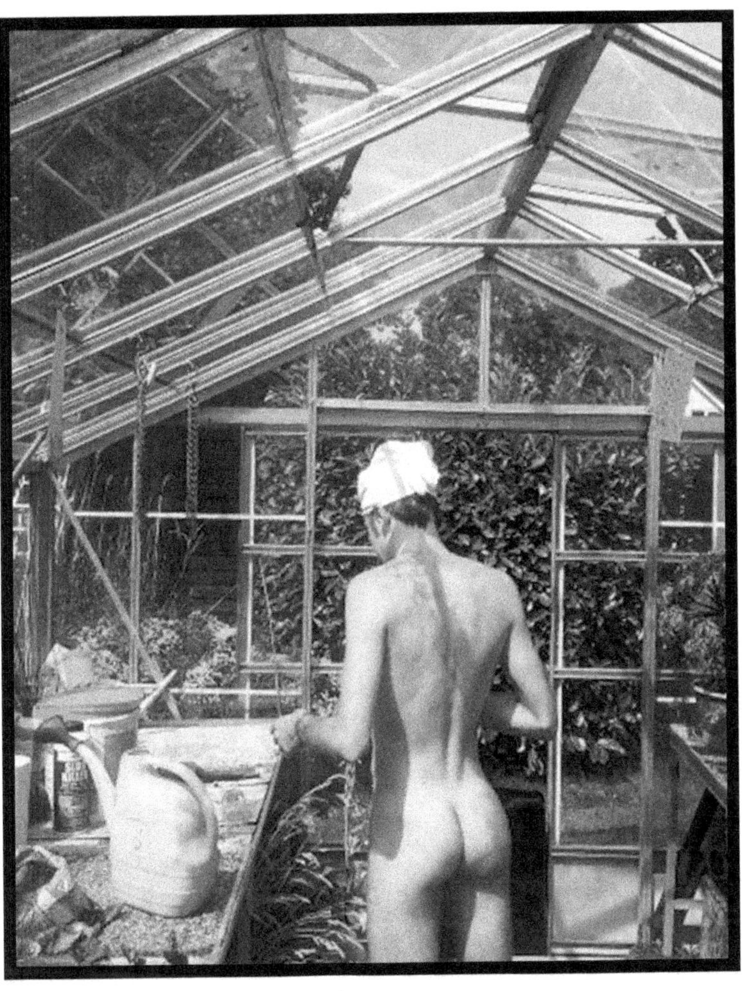

I know a few people who garden and do yard work nude as well. Gardening nude can be dirty, but your skin washes off easier than clothes, plus similarly to exercising, it allows you to sweat naturally and keep cool. It should go without saying, if it's illegal to be outside naked where you live, don't do it.

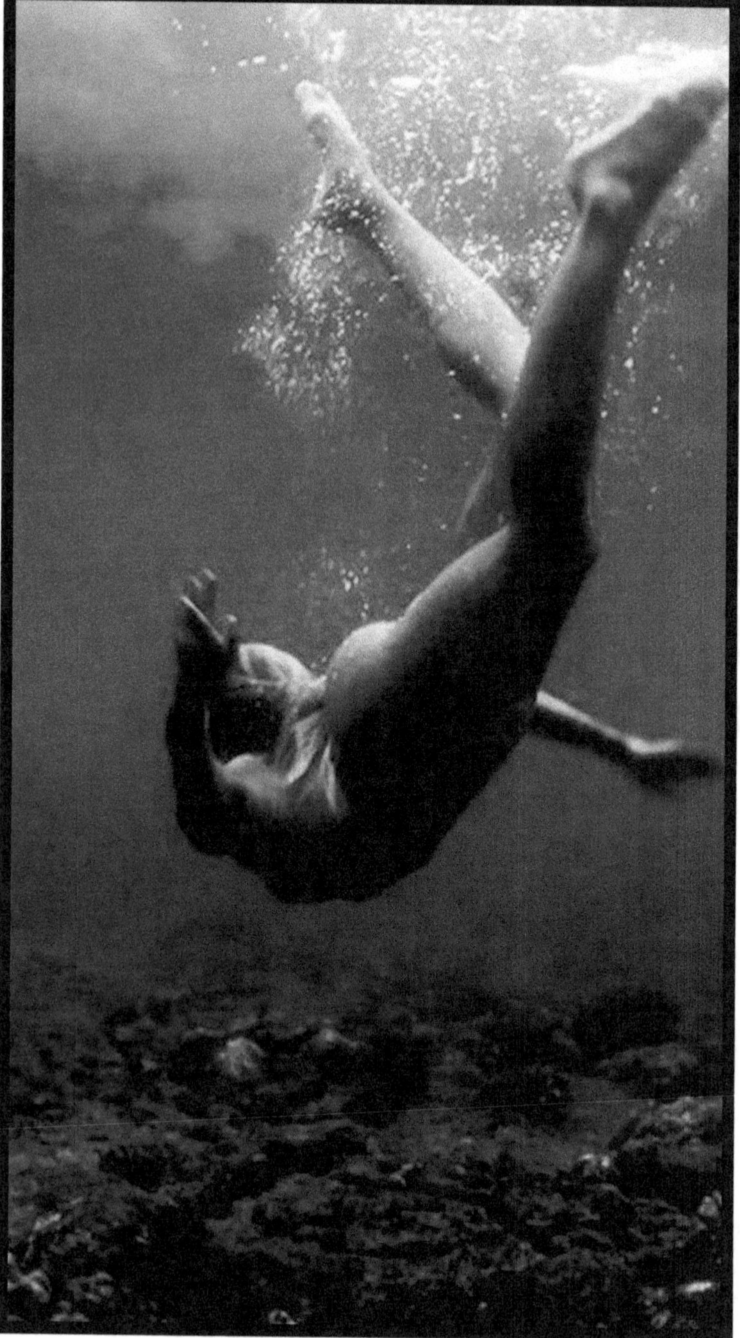

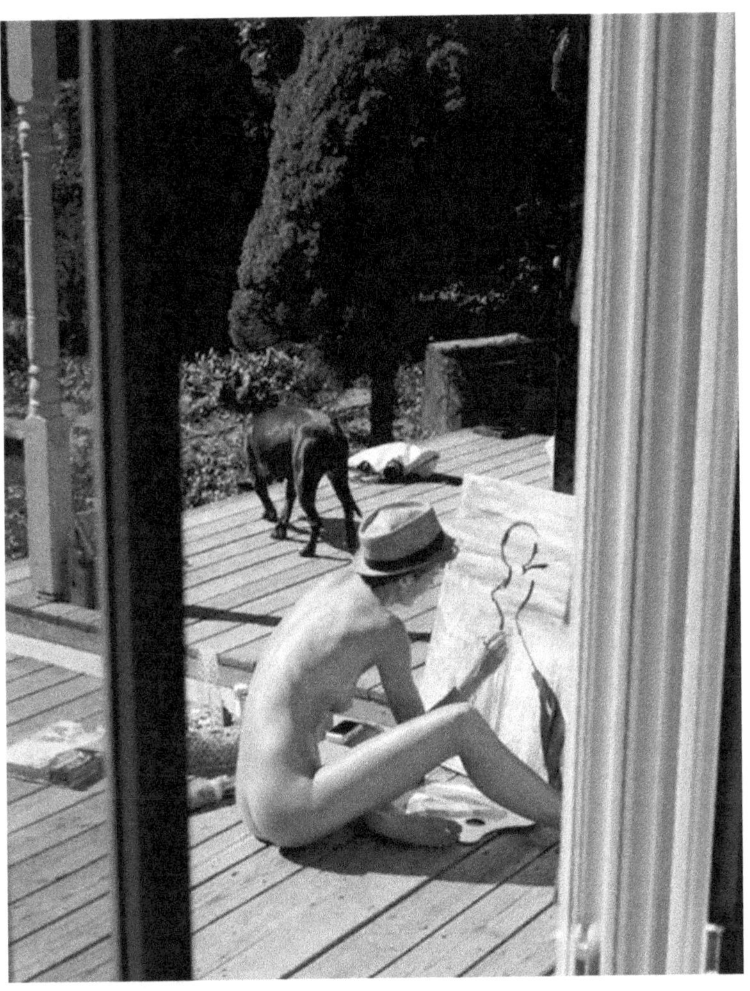

If this is the case, you can stick to indoor activities, like painting or simple home repairs. There are lots of people who paint nude to protect their clothes, since paint wont stain your skin permanently.

We've gone over cooking and cleaning nude, and even some work around the house. But if you work from home, why not do that too?

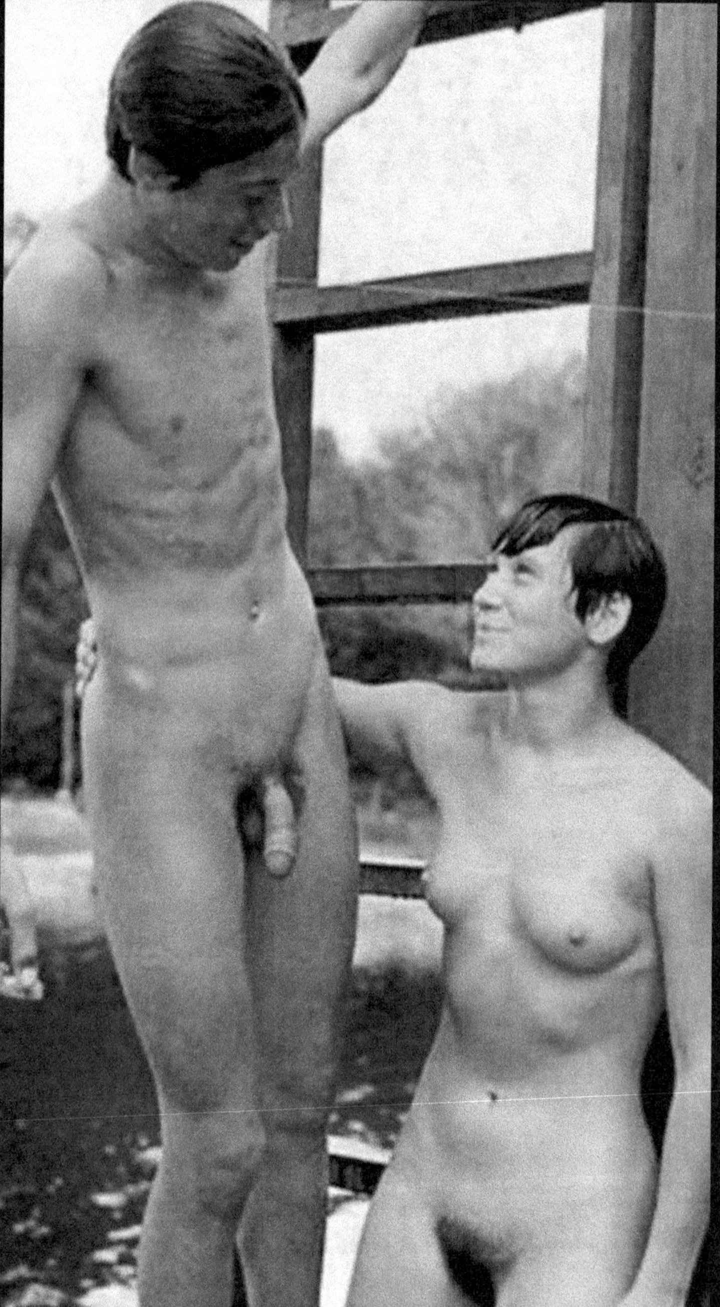

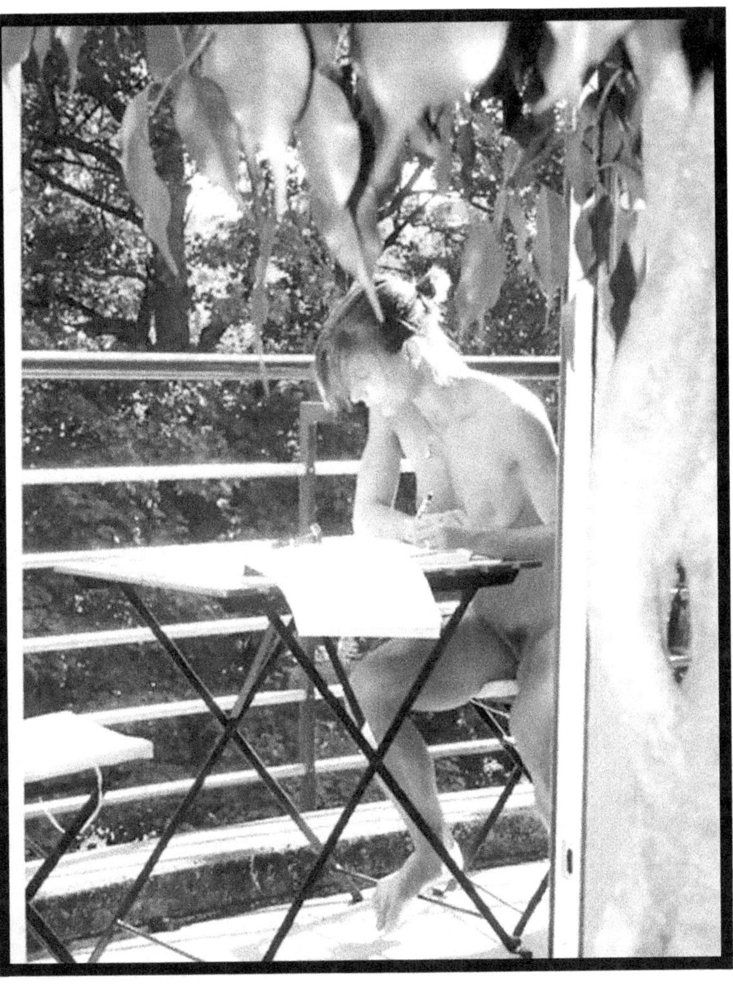

I have witnessed people that, for their profession, they are required to make video calls from their home office, and in these events, they have put on a button down shirt and tie, but are still naked from the waist down. Why not? No one can see anyway right?

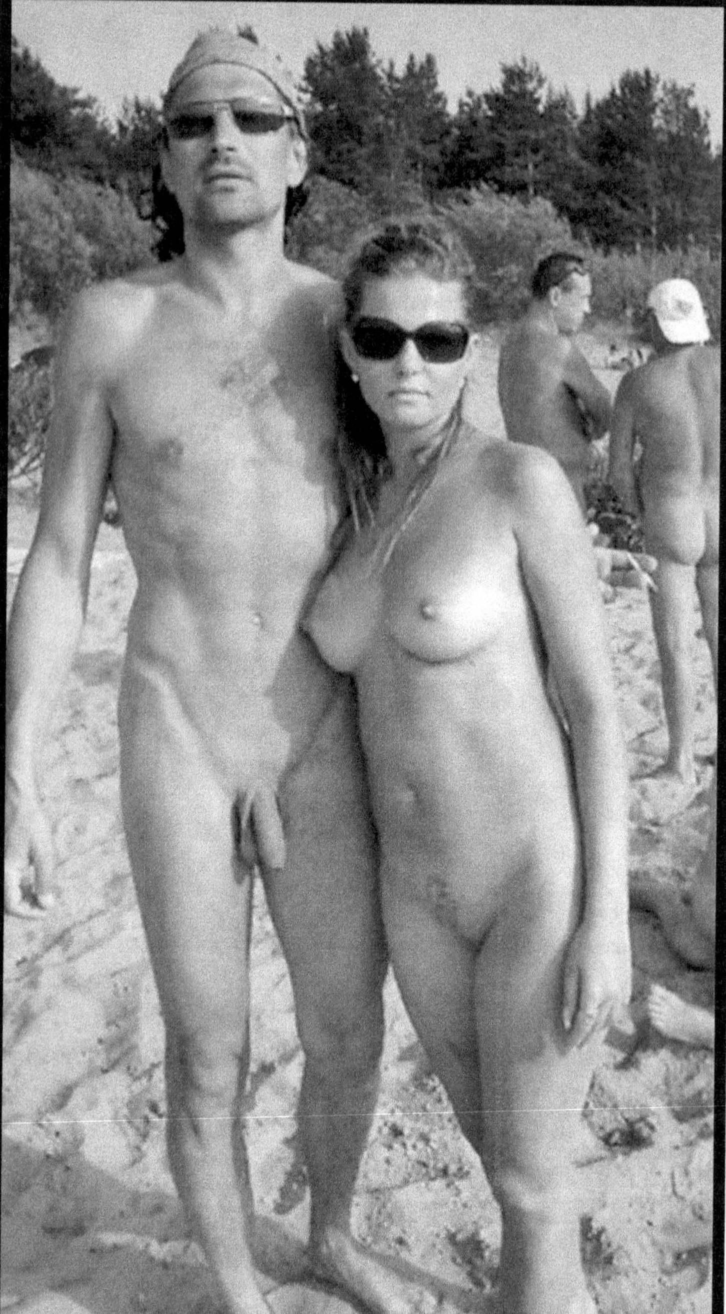

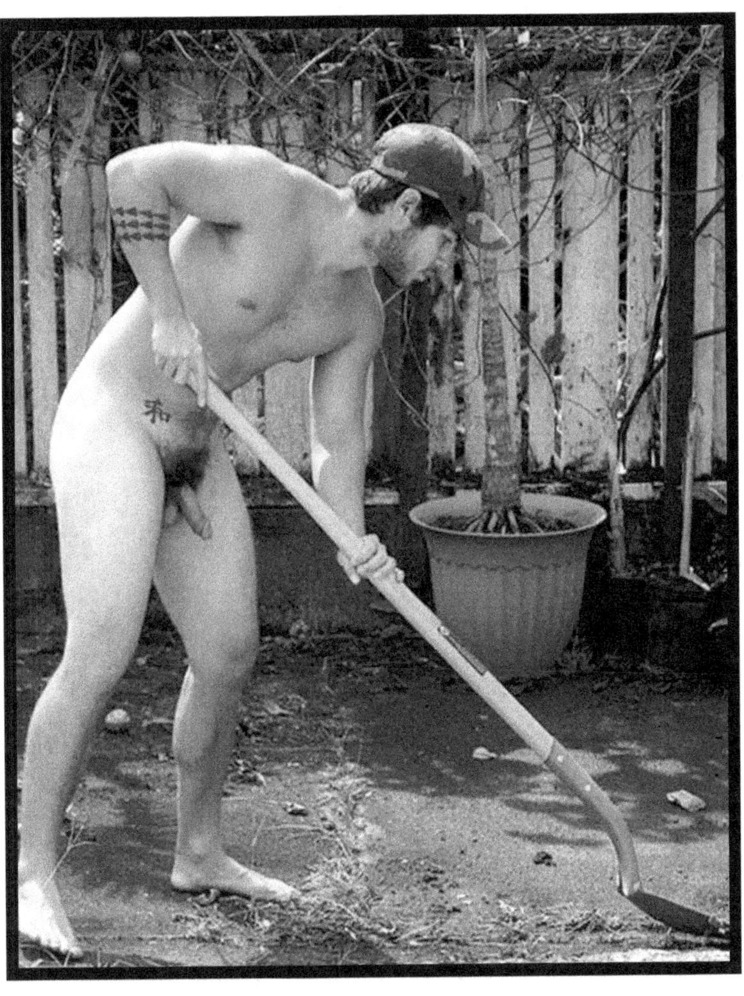

To summarize this idea, why should your daily life at home be any different because you're nude? Whether you live alone or have a spouse and kids, there's no reason we cannot be comfortable in our own homes.

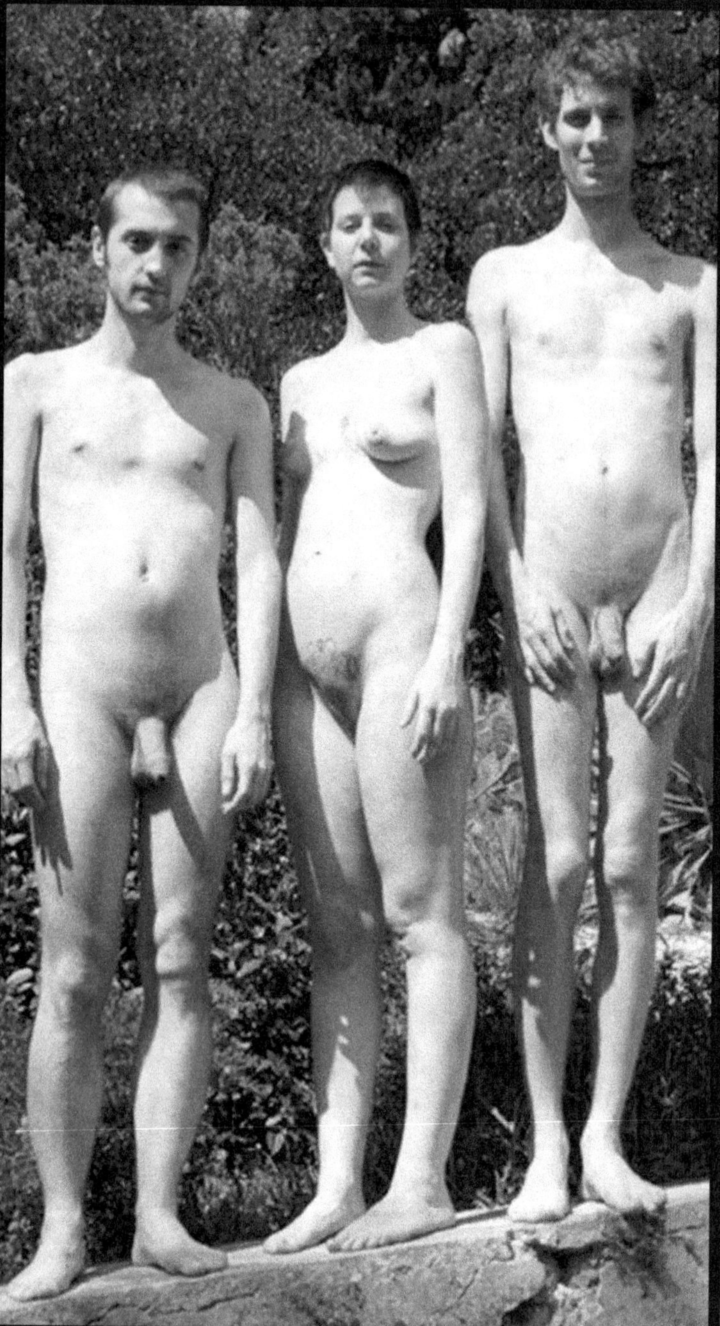

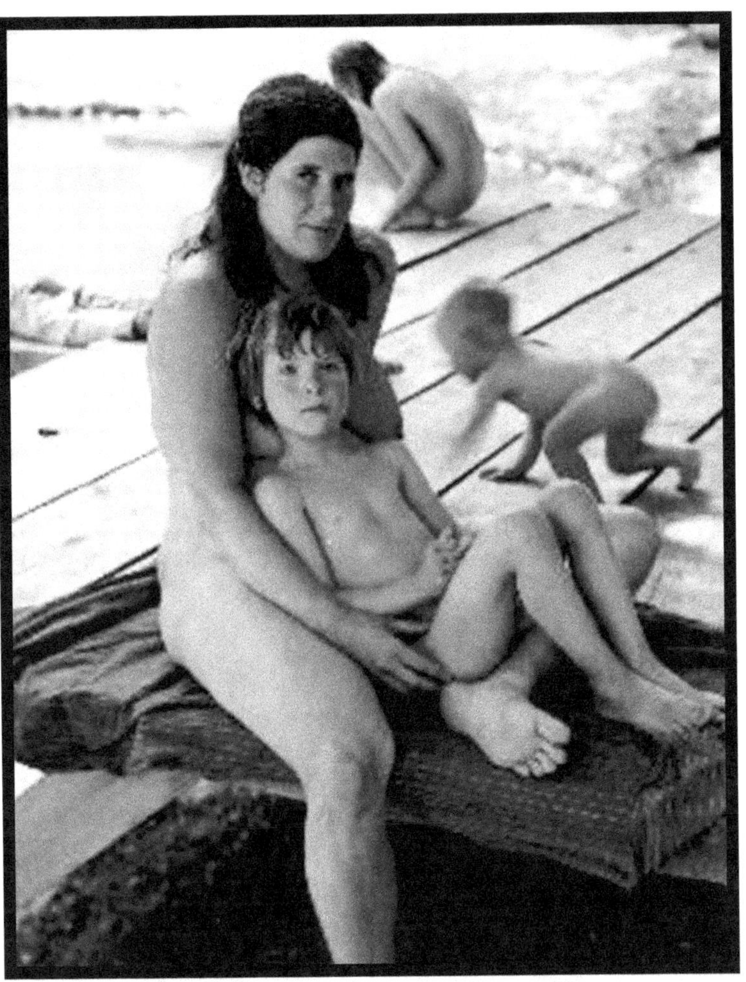

Raising a Nude Family

I have heard many people argue that it is inappropriate for kids and parents to be naked all the time and that it is unhealthy for the kids. I would argue that it is actually healthier than not raising them nude.

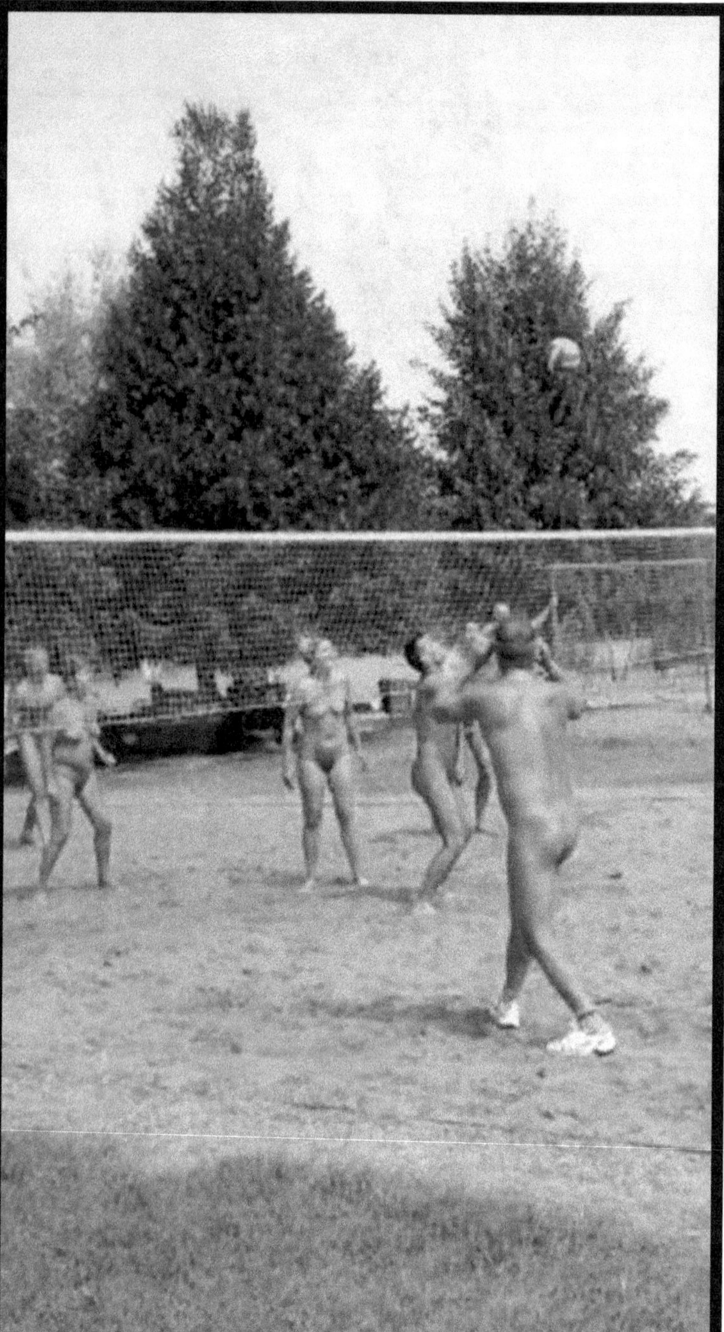

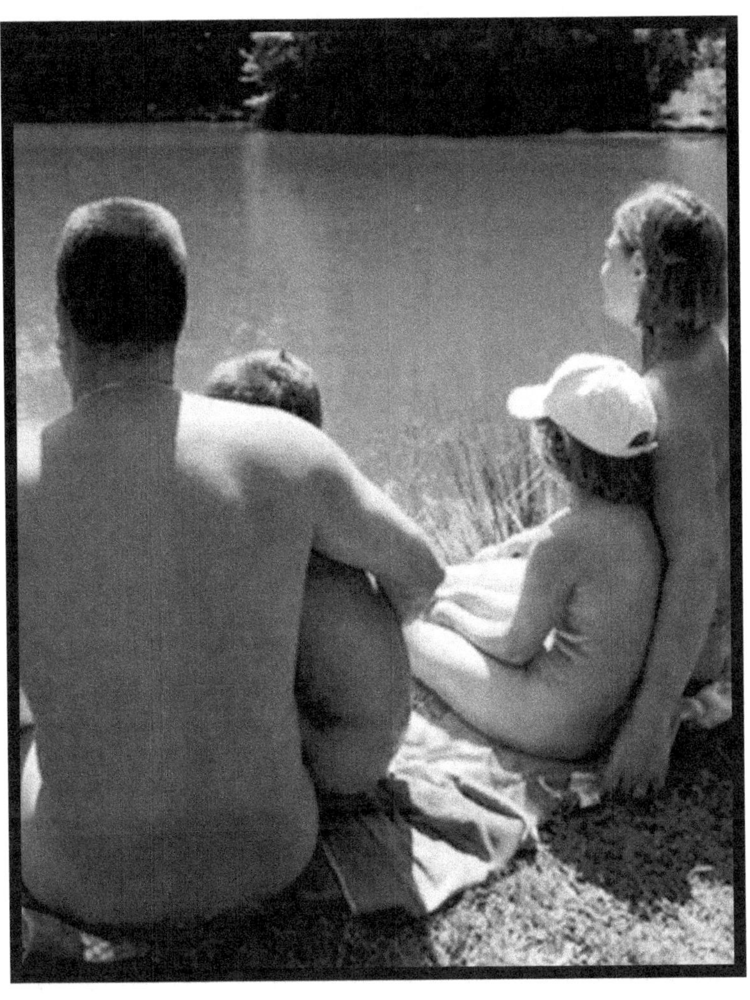

Like with anything that we teach our kids, there has to be some time spent teaching the opposite view point as well. The last thing you want is your elementary school child going to school and just stripping down in class. And you also don't want them to feel ashamed either.

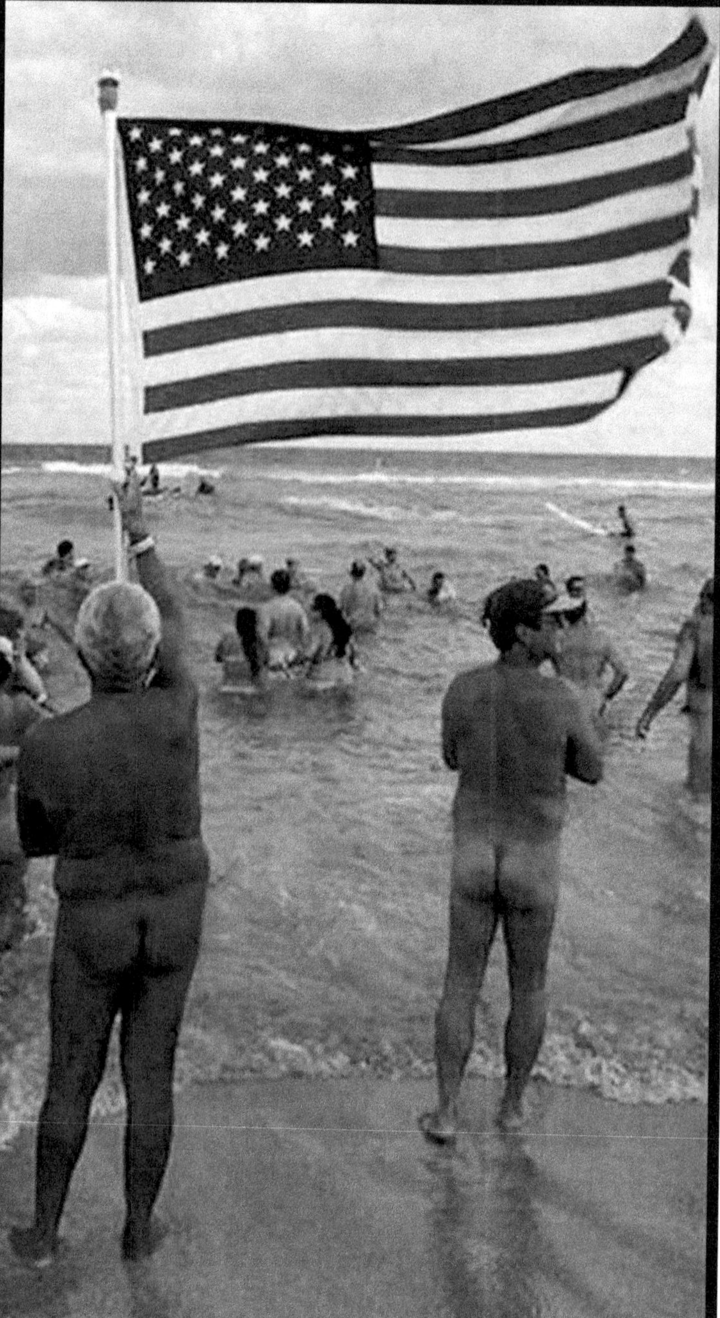

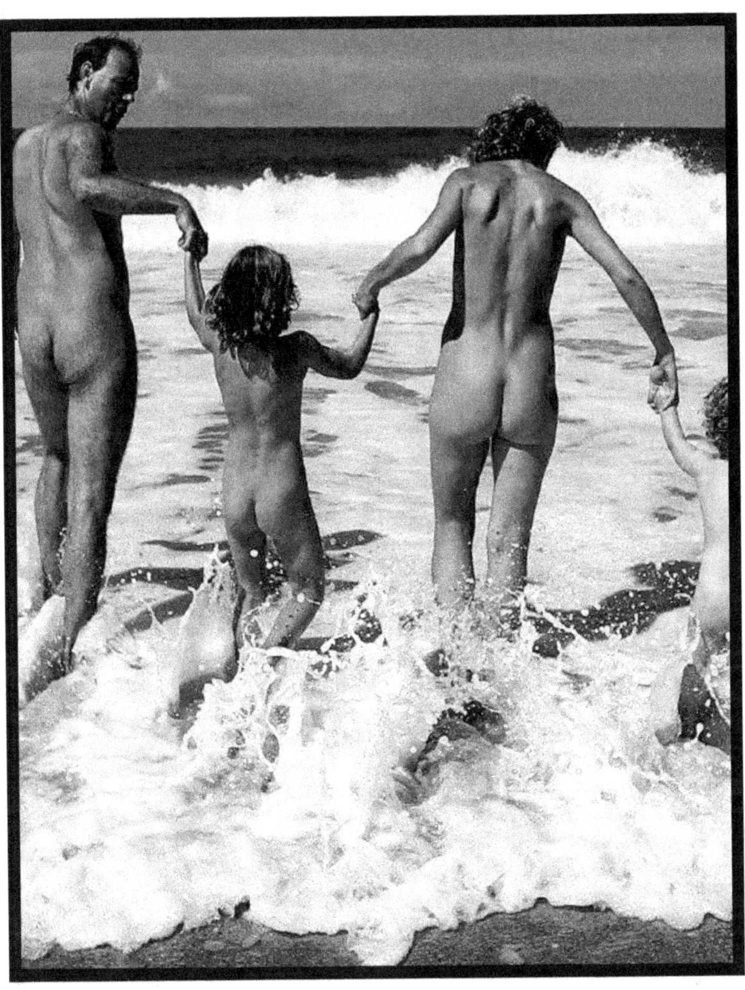

Teaching your kids at an early age why nudism is normal is important, but it is also important to teach them why people who wear clothes all day is also normal. Another key thing is to make sure your kids understand that they have a choice in the matter.

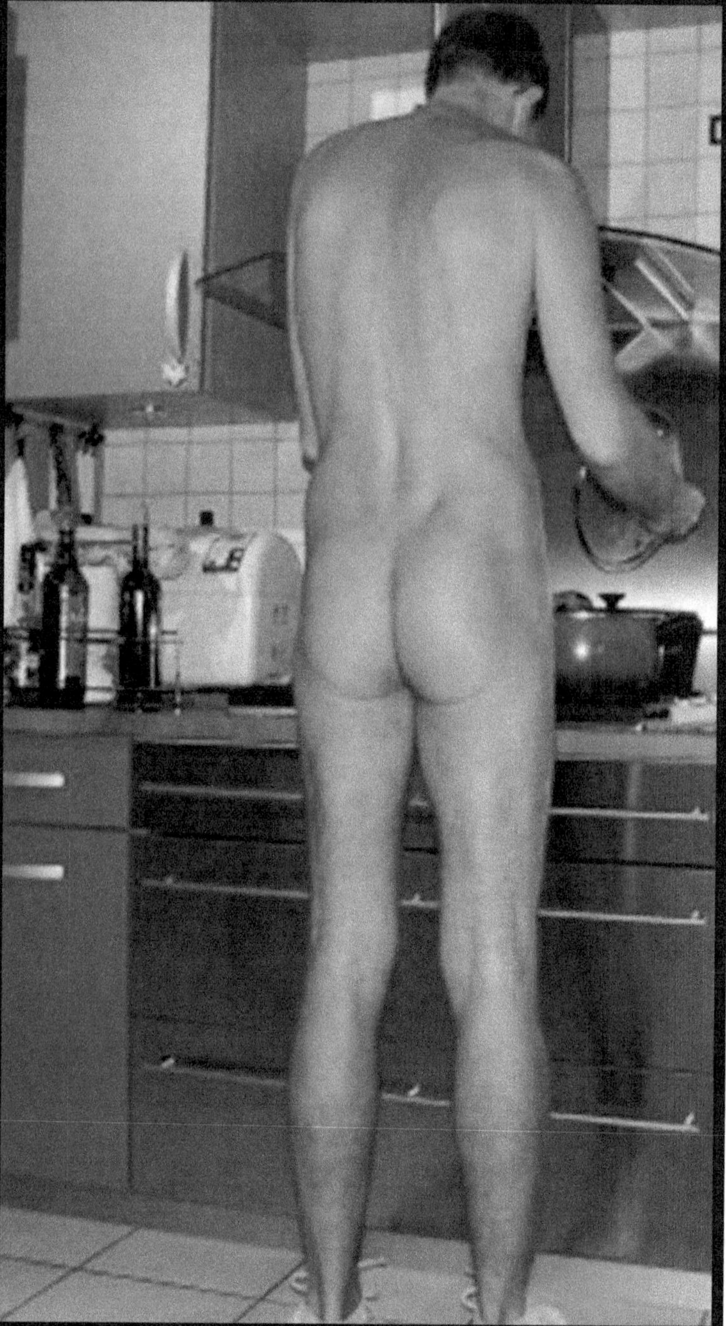

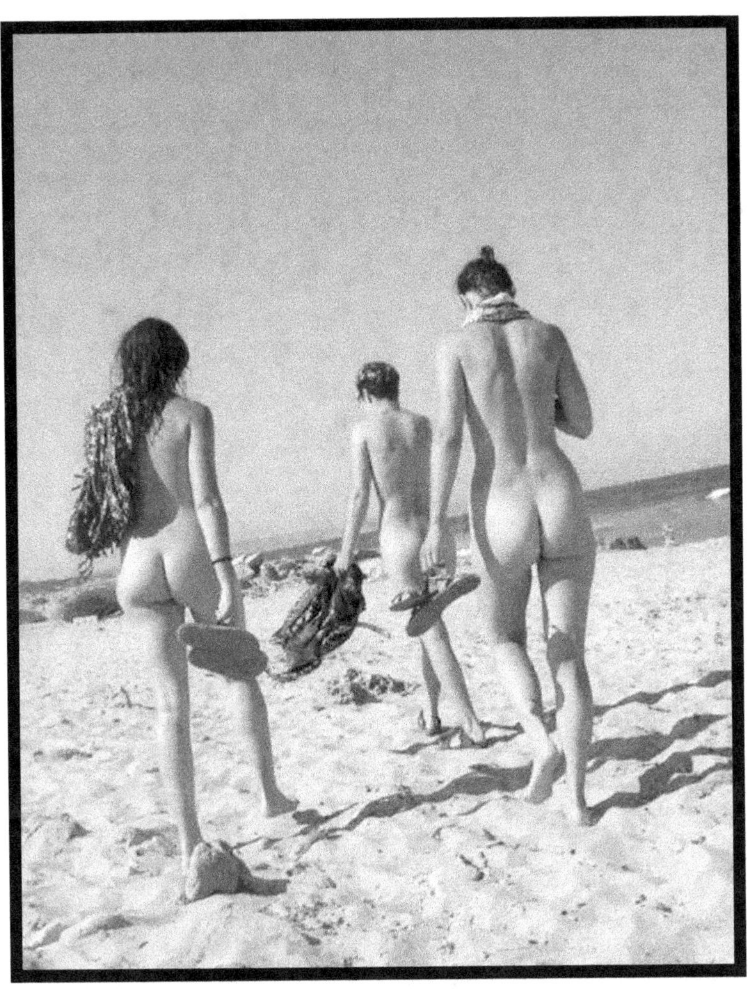

While you may require them to be nude at home, at least in certain circumstances it may be a good idea to give them the option as well. For example, I had the idea of doing a "Nude Tuesday," where we only are naked on weekends and Tuesdays.

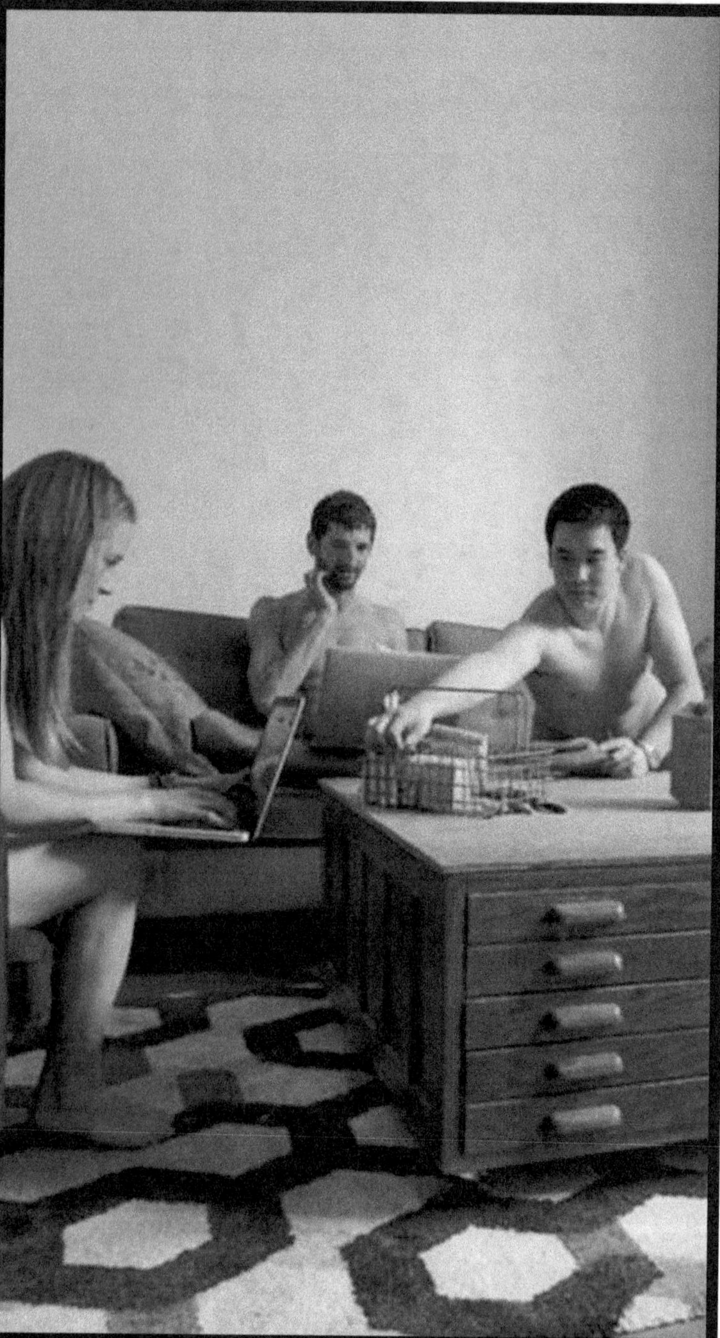

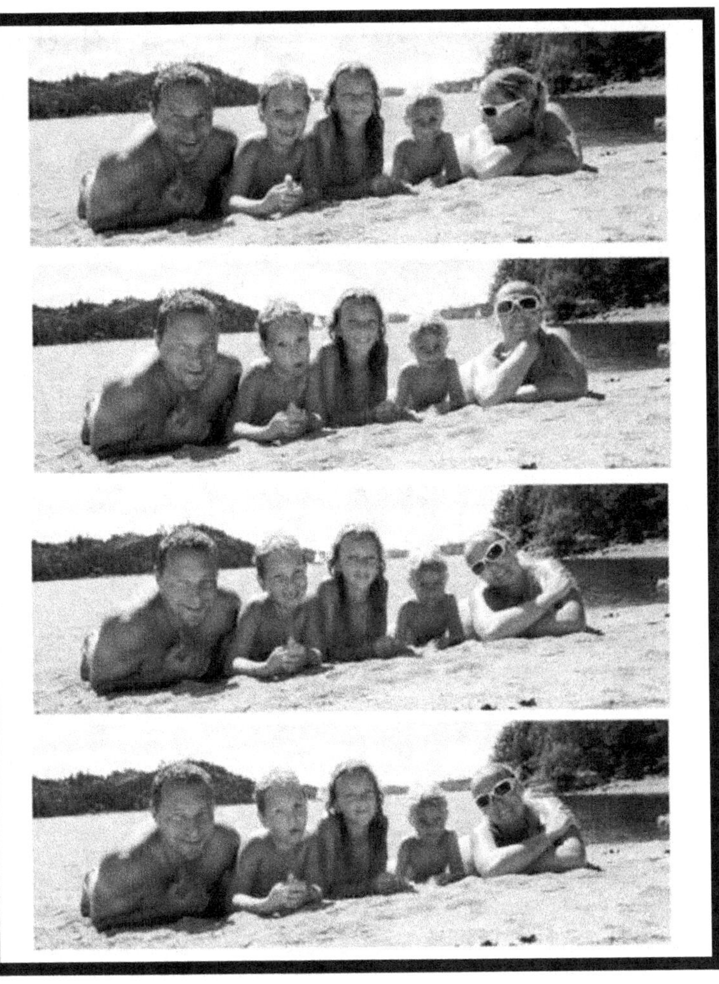

Allowing some freedom to choose will help the child realize that nudism either is or isn't for them, without the pressure that we, as nudists, are trying to avoid from people that wear clothes every day.

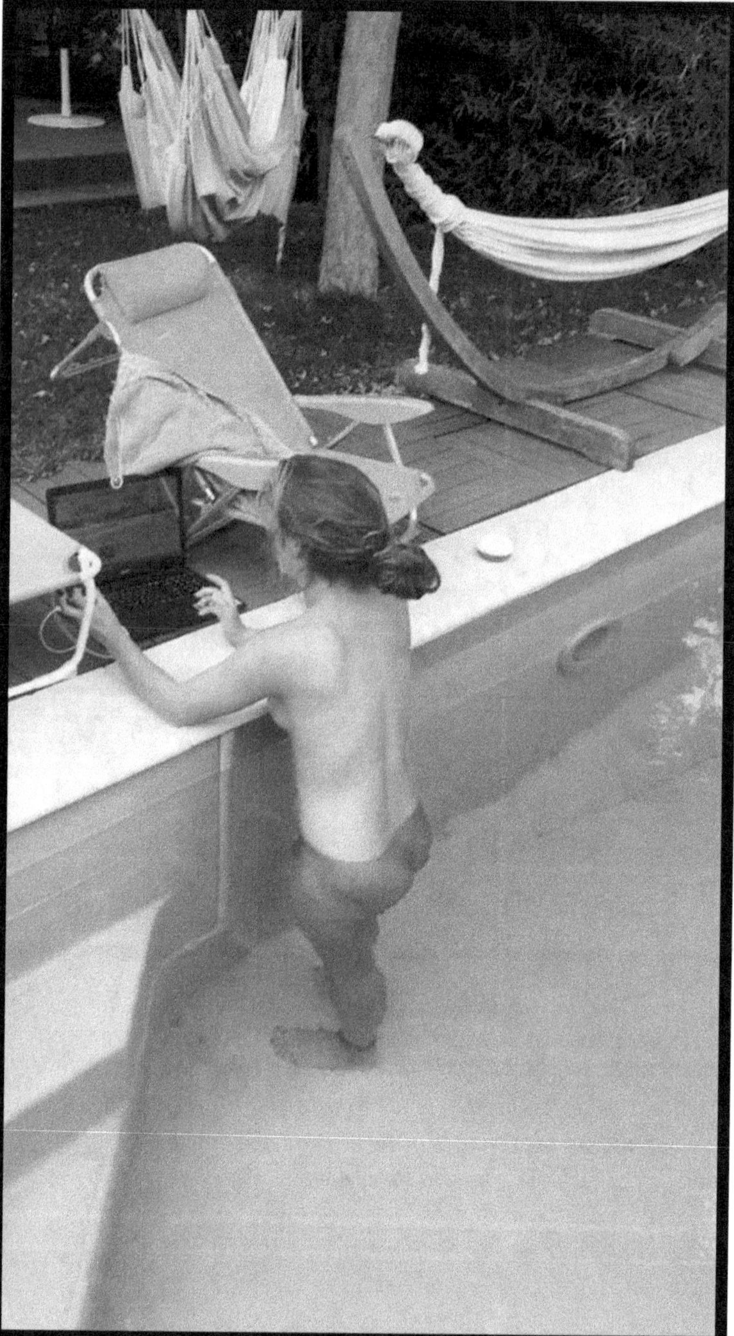

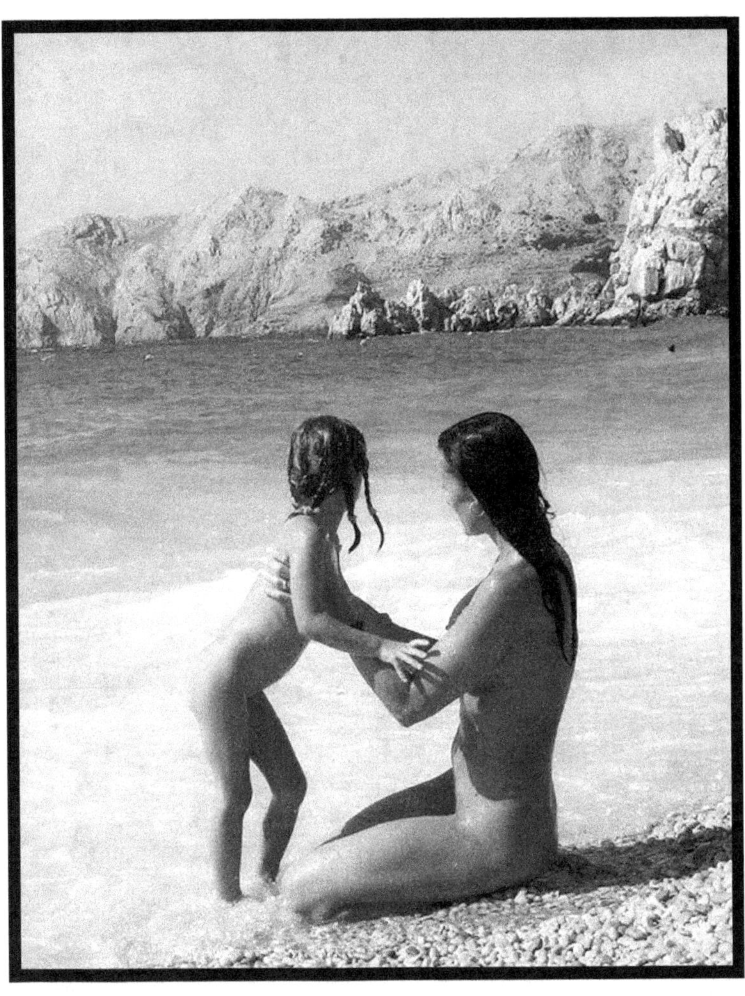

So how does being nude help the child? Well for one, it reduces clothes that need to be washed, and I am sure anyone with small children understands why this would be a blessing. However, there are a lot more benefits than that.

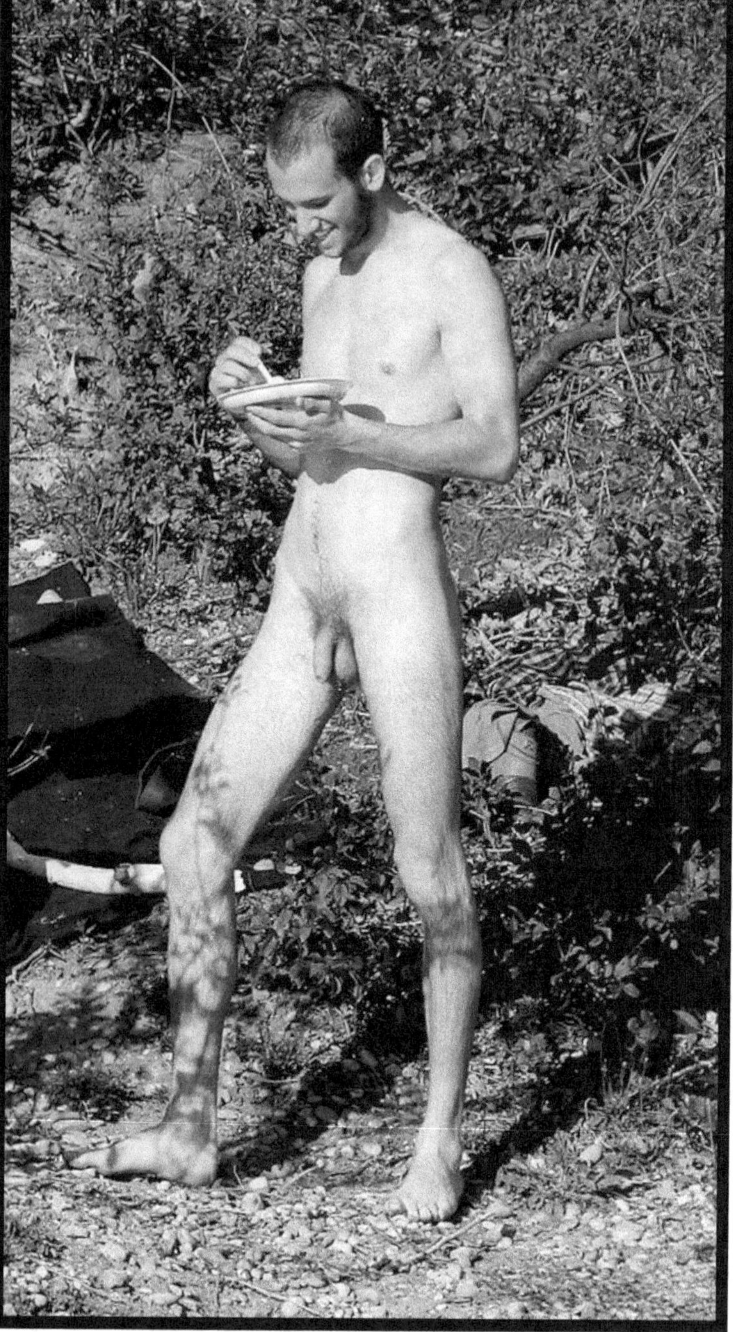

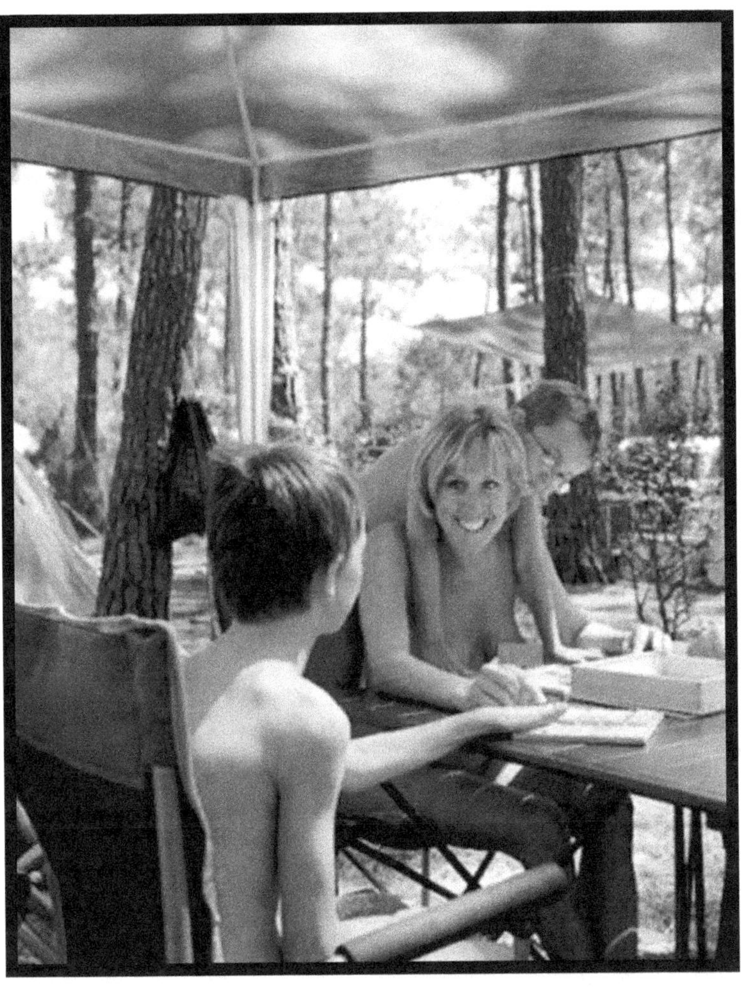

The biggest benefit would be the increase in self-esteem. As a child grows and goes through puberty, their body changes, and if most adults think back, that is when we really started to feel self-conscious about our bodies.

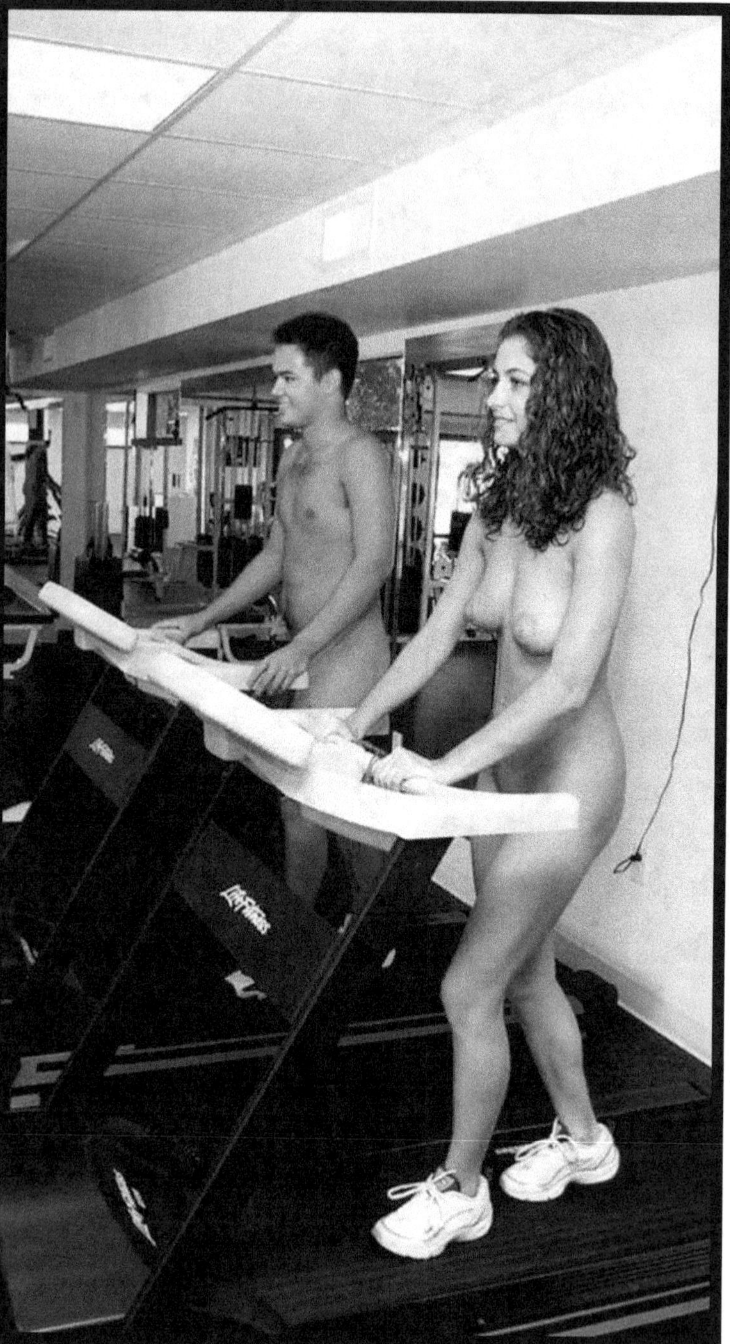

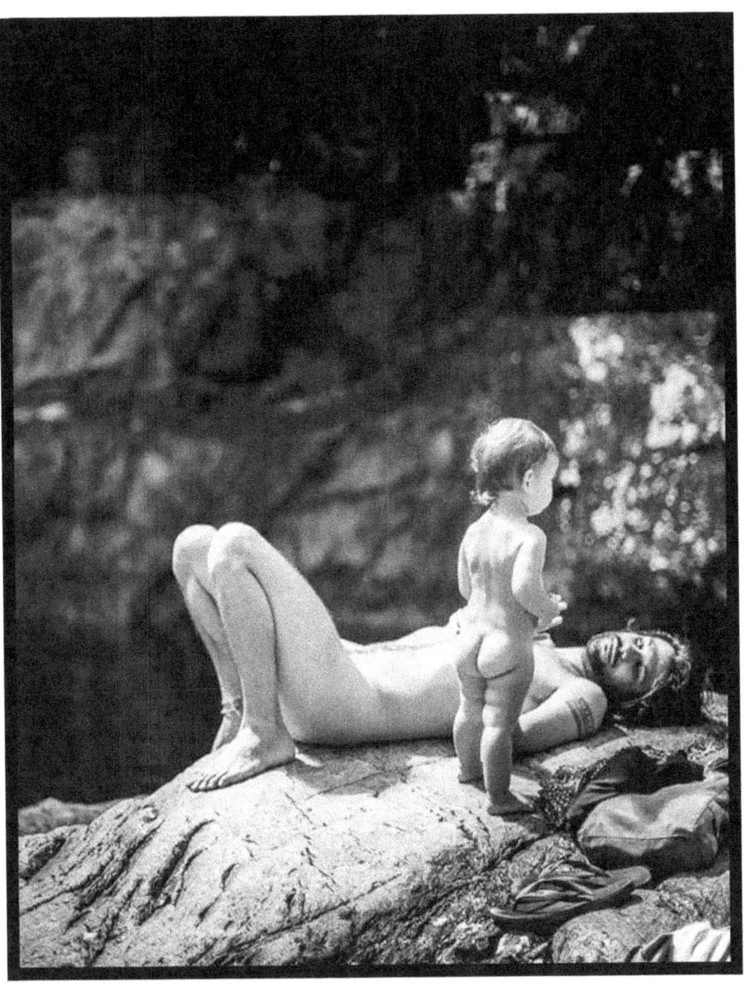

Because no one is hiding the features of their body, a child has nothing to be ashamed of, as hair begins to grow in places or parts start to change in size and shape, they will see that this is normal.
Also, with a child that has been exposed to nudity at a young age, there is no real reason to objectify a human body, it's normal for a young boy to see a naked girl and vice versa.

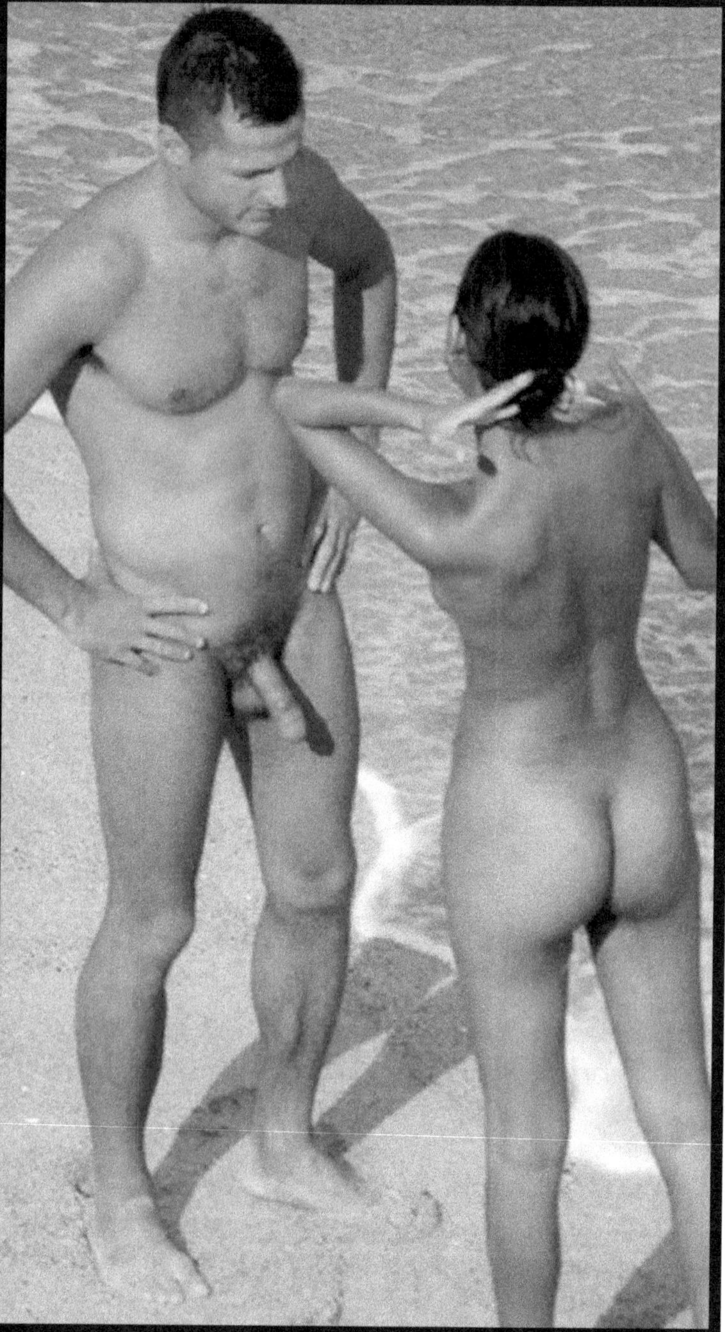

This concludes our introduction book. If you would like more information, check out some of my other titles that are a more in depth guide to nudism.

Just a few parting notes, I am not the photographer or owner of the photos in this book, they were acquired through open source websites and as such fall under the category of public images. If you desire to use them for your own purposes, feel free to do so at your leisure.

However, the information and wording in this book are my own, and therefore I ask that you request my permission before using or quoting any part of my work.

Thanks again for reading.

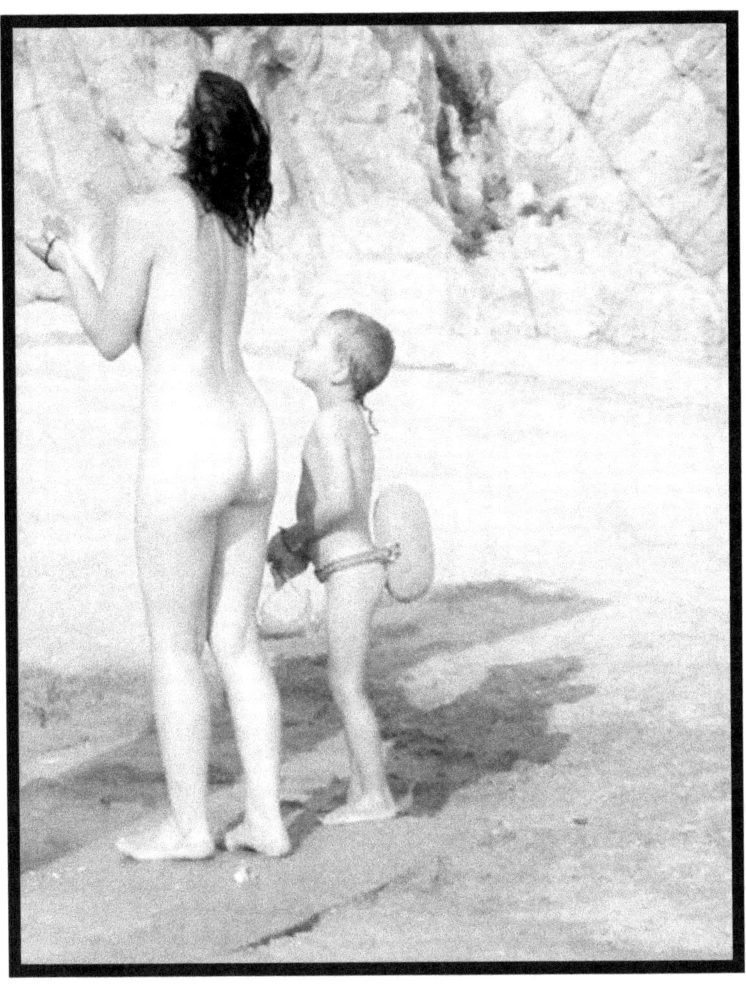

Of course boys still have hormones and will get an erection from time to time, but this is normal and natural. The best advice I have read is to just act normal and not make a big deal out of it.

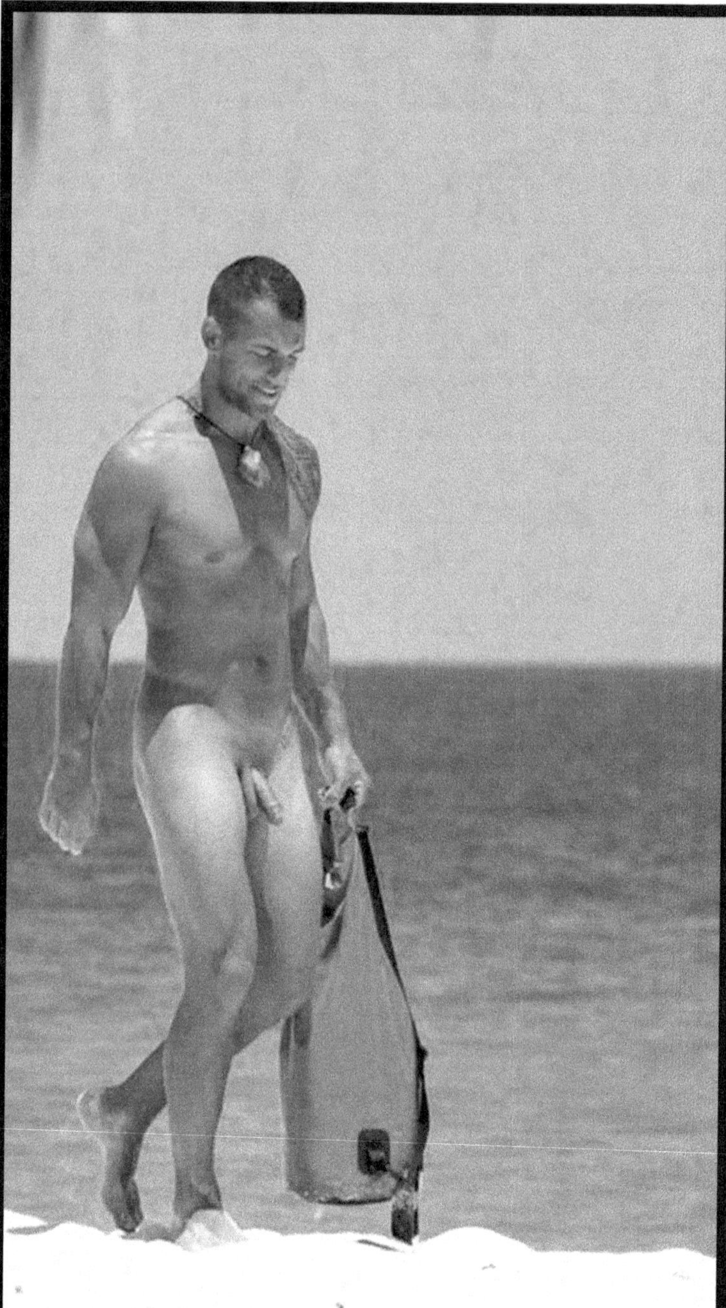

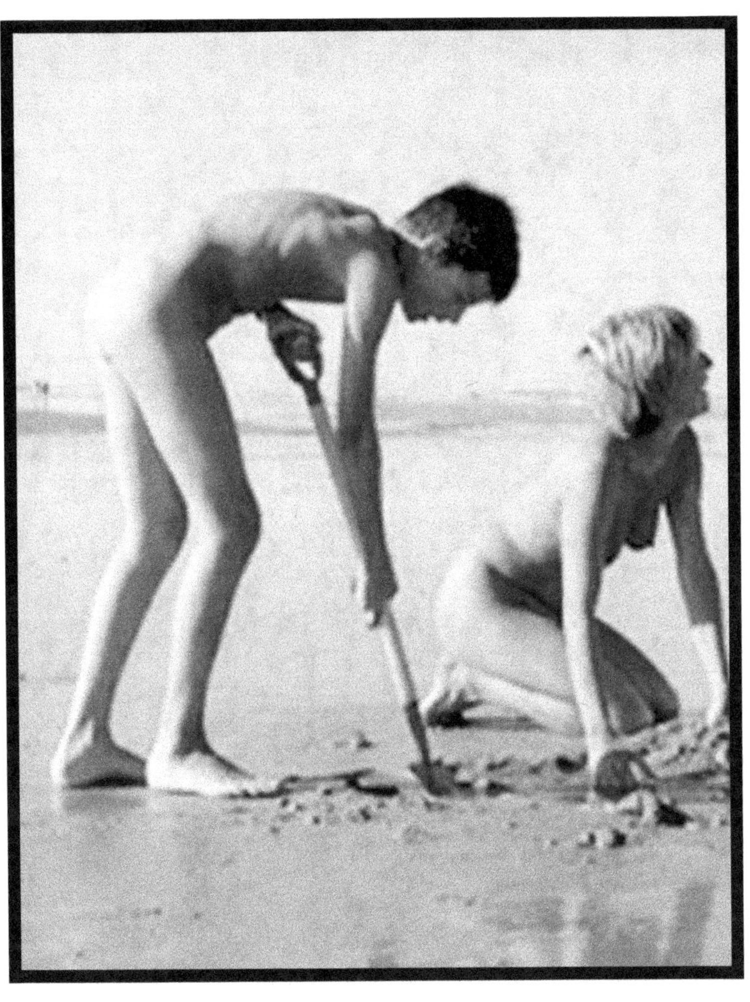

Now, going back to your child and socializing with others. Obviously not all of your child's friends, if any, will be from nudist families, and again, you should teach your child this from an early age. There are a couple options when it comes to dealing with this situation as a parent.

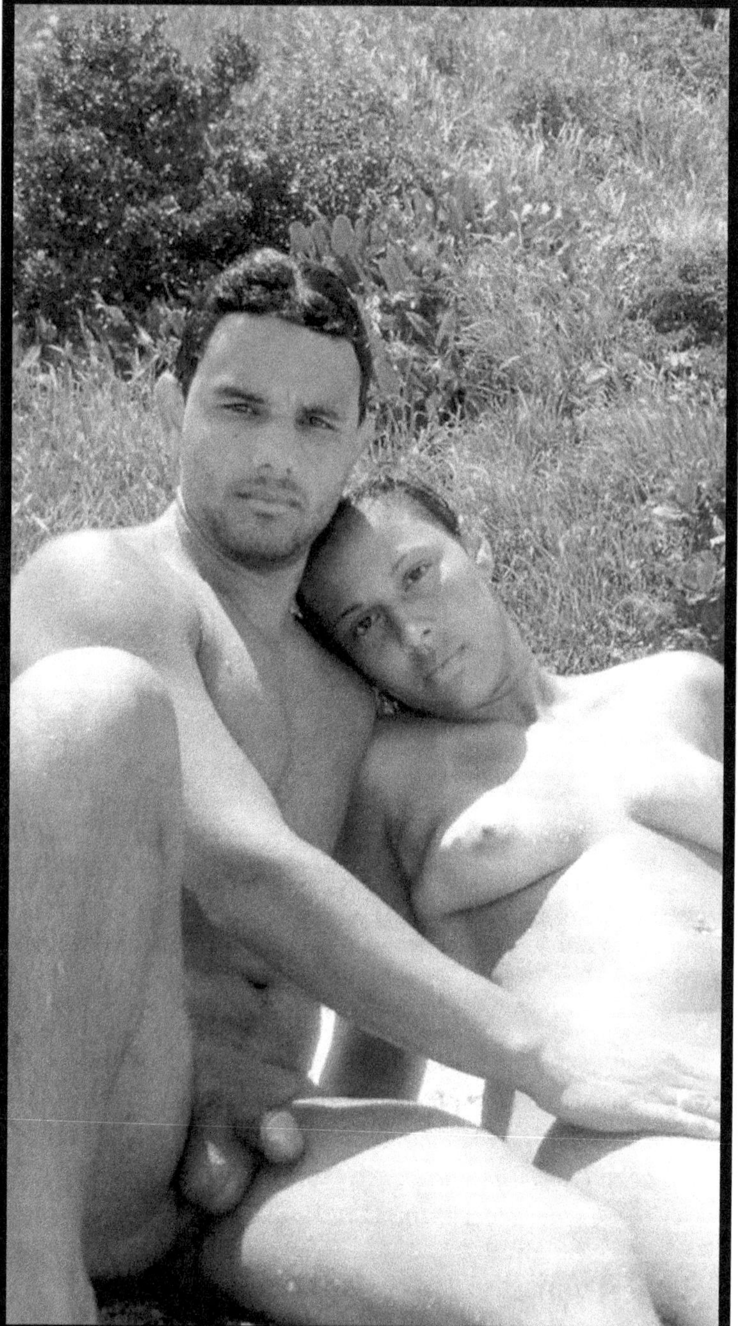

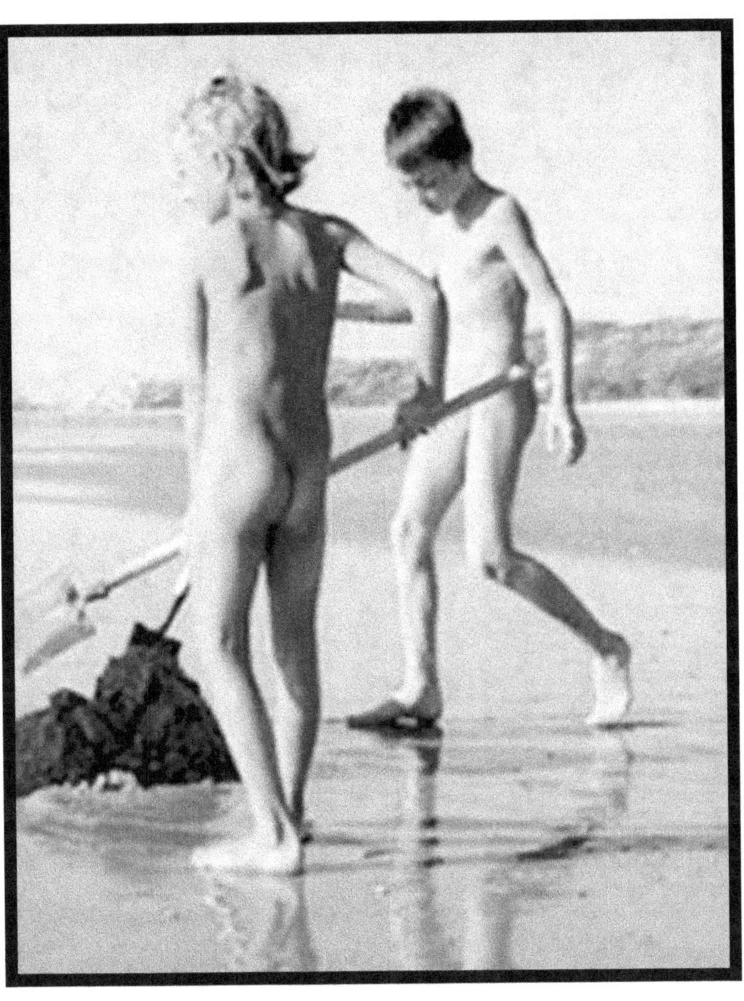

If you are comfortable with the idea, perhaps the best way to approach the issue is to take some time and talk to the parents of the other kid. Explain what nudism is and why you and your family partake in it. At that point, give the other child's parents the choice of whether they want their child in that environment or not.

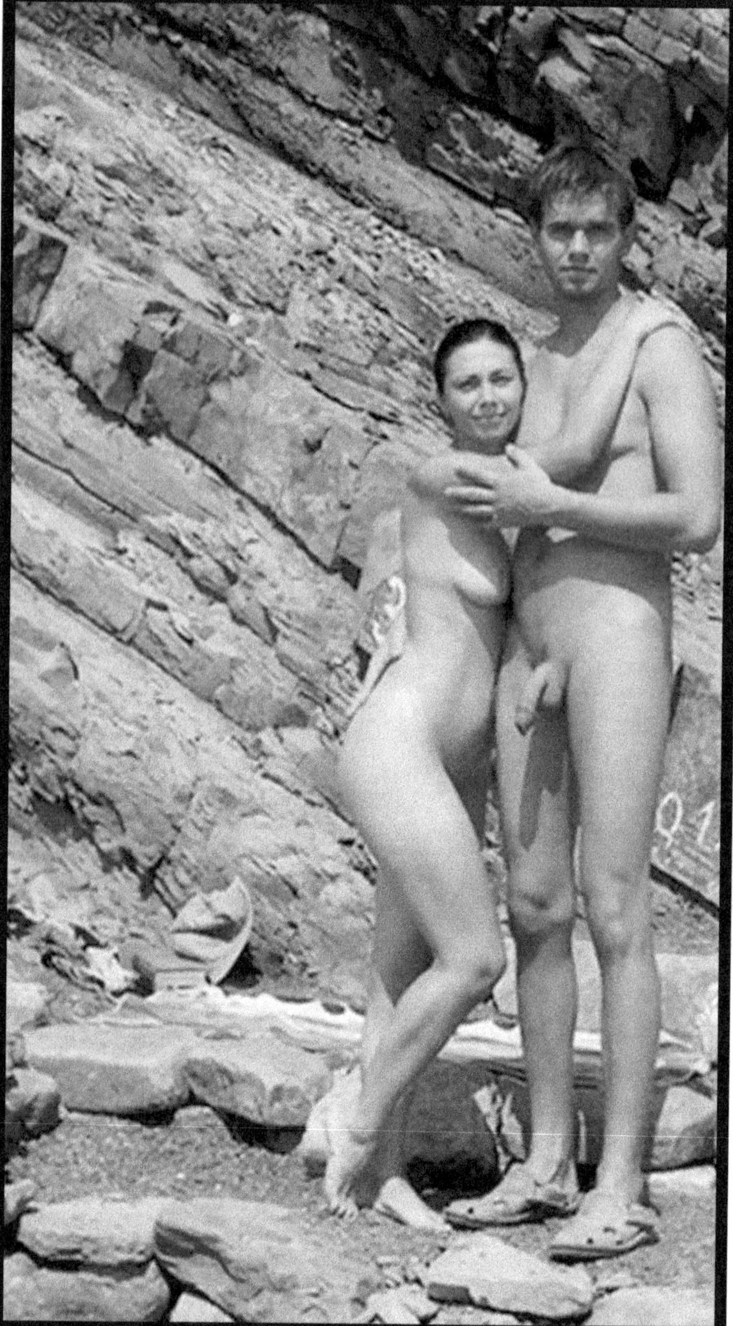

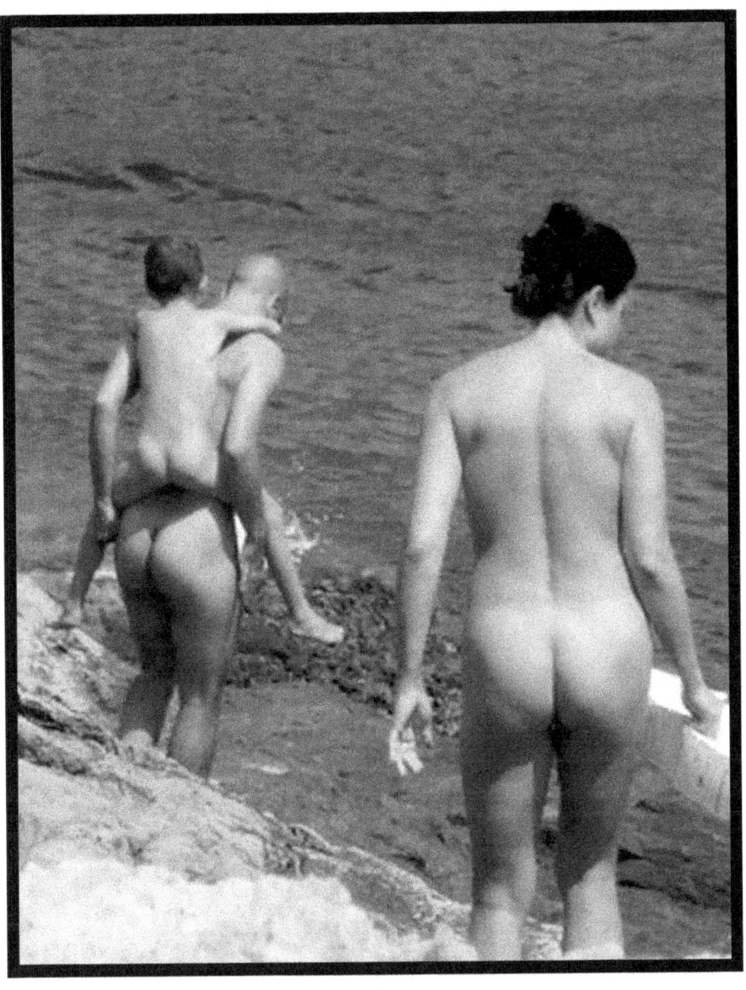

If they say that their child is fine in that environment, maybe invite the parents over for an adult only nudist dinner party or something similar, and see if they would be interested in partaking as well. Or if they seem opposed to the idea of nudism, perhaps you would compromise and keep your family clothed while their child is at your house.

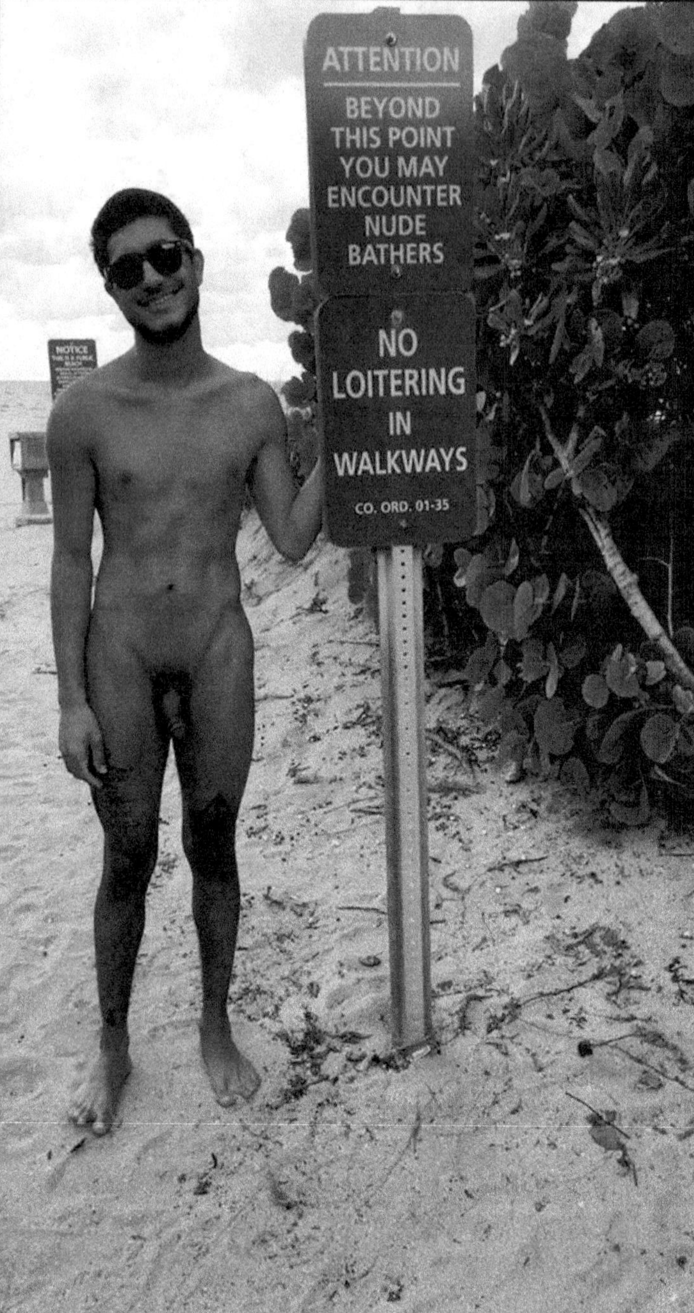

ATTENTION
BEYOND
THIS POINT
YOU MAY
ENCOUNTER
NUDE
BATHERS
NO
LOITERING
IN
WALKWAYS
CO. ORD. 01-35
NOTICE
THIS IS A PUBLIC
BEACH

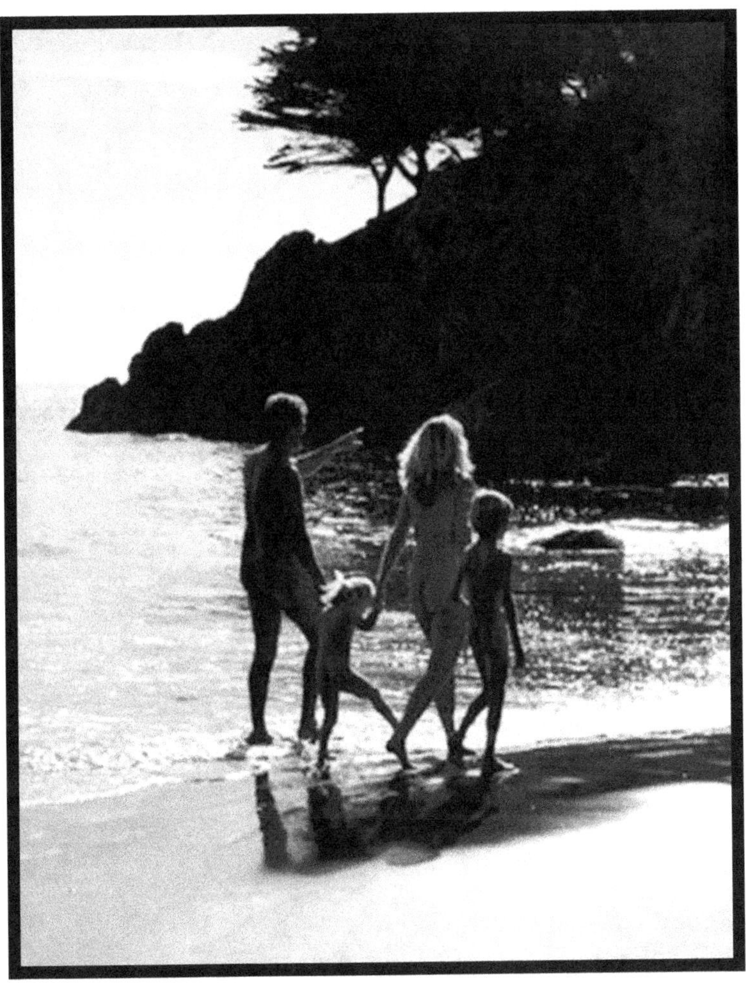

The other option that you have as a parent is to just have your family get dressed before you have any company over. This may be the best option in a lot of situations where the majority of the neighbors seem closed minded, or if you do not wish to let your neighbors know of your lifestyle. Your child may prefer this option, so I would leave the choice up to them, if at all possible.

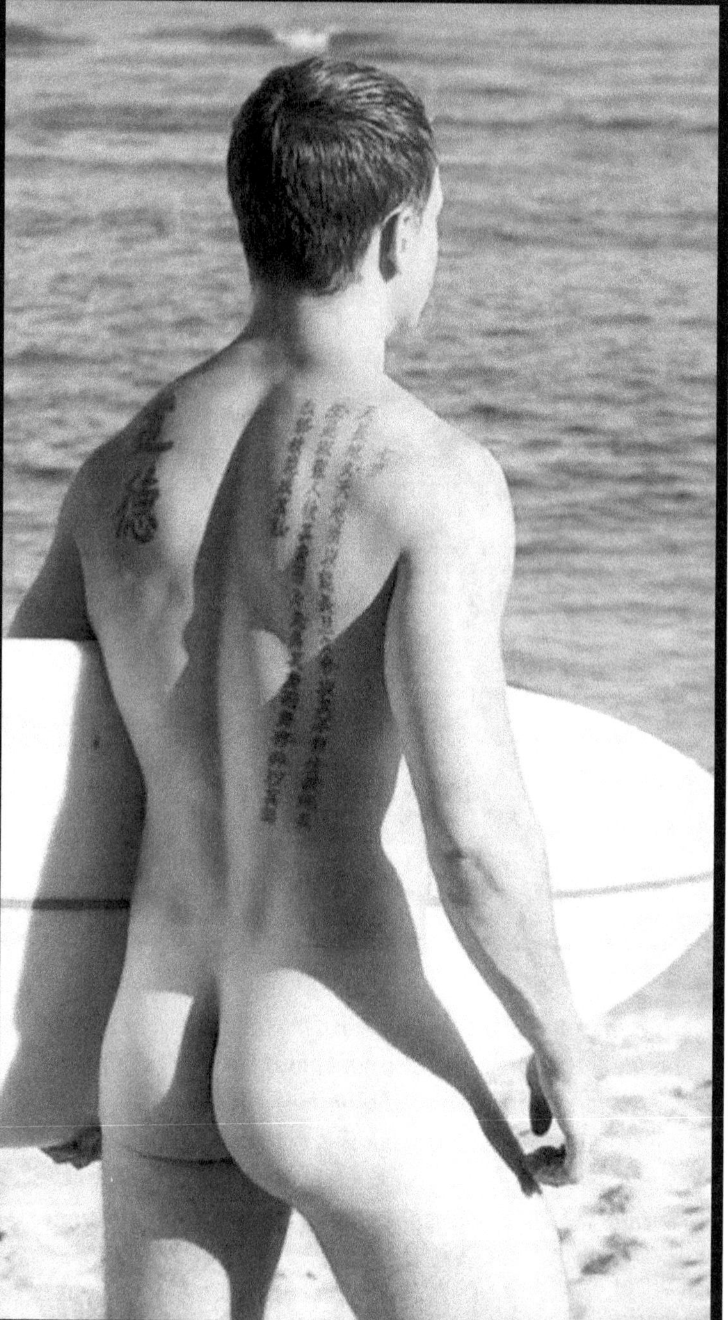

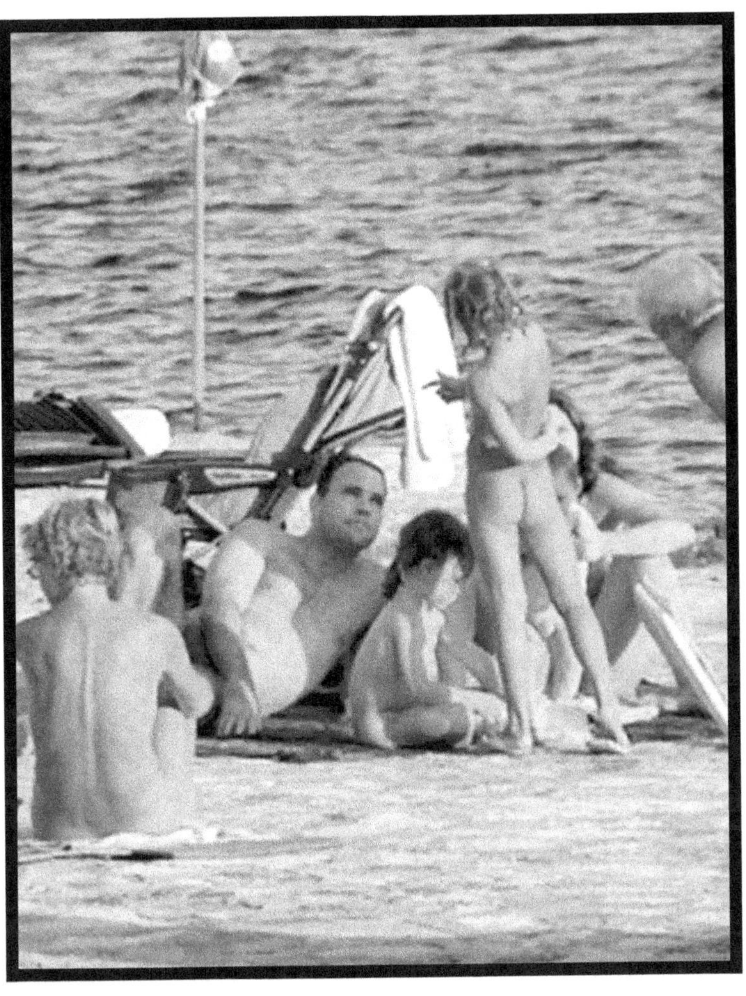

One study that I read stated, "The viewing of the unclothed body, far from being destructive to the psyche, seems to be either benign and totally harmless or to actually provide benefits to the individual involved."

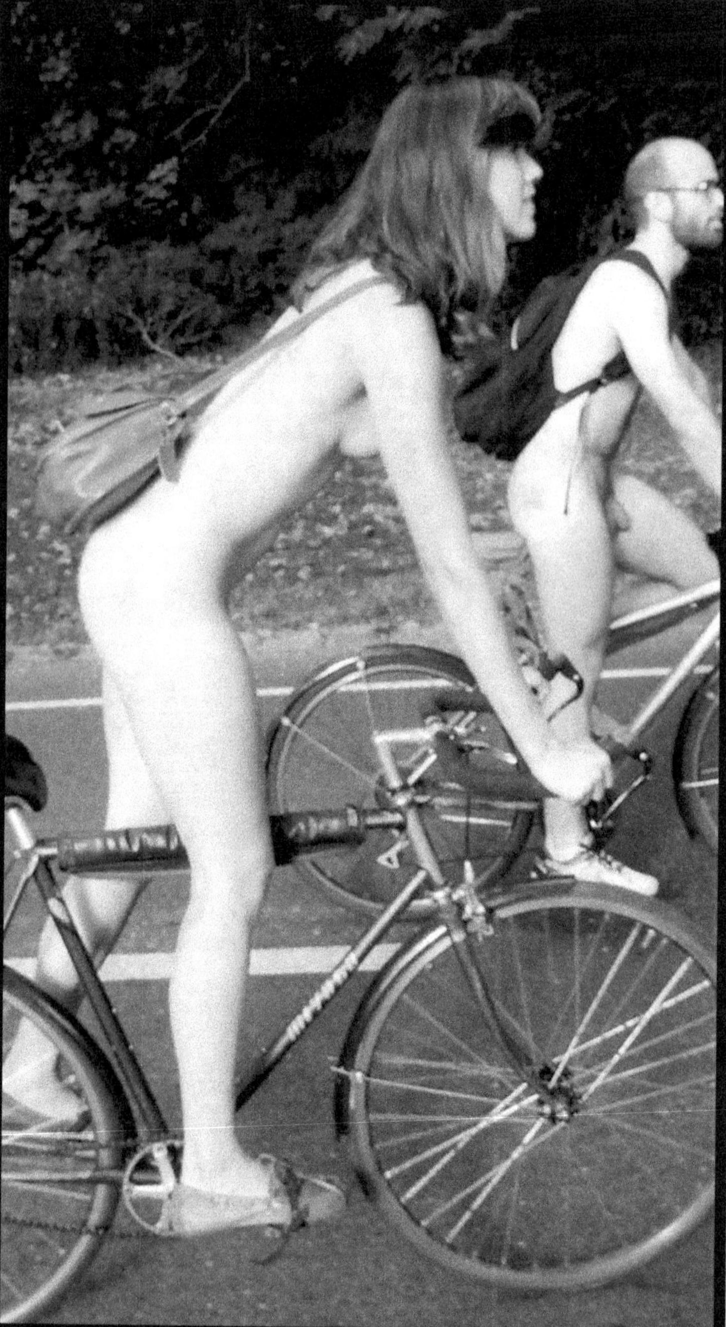

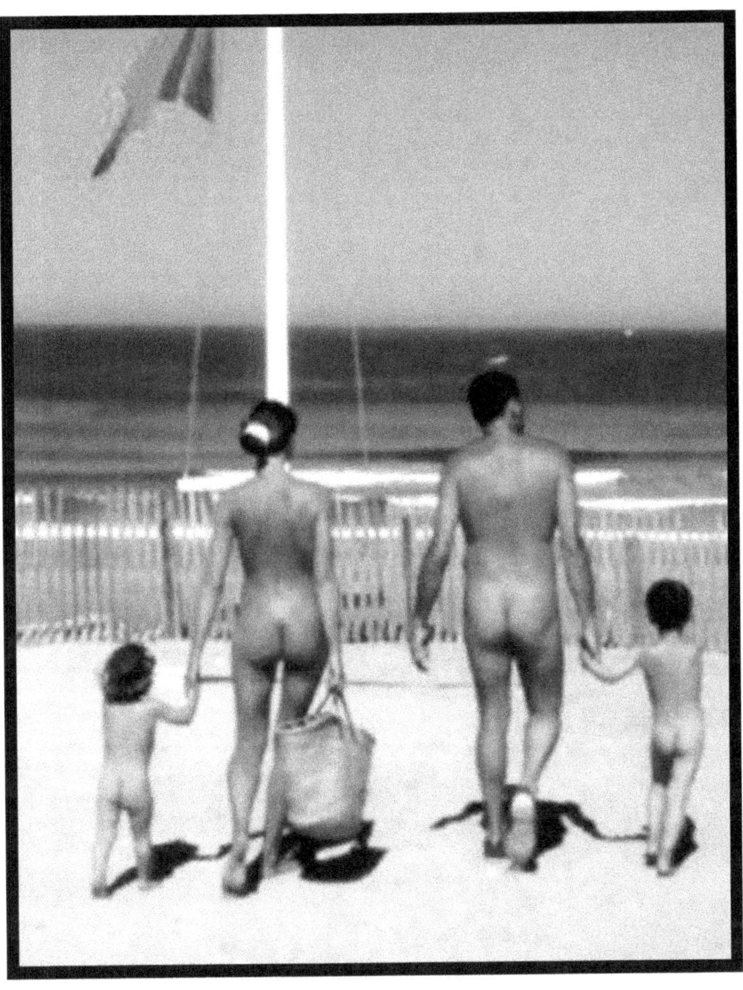

So like with living a nude life, why not raise a nude family? Studies have proven that either the child has a stronger self-image, which leads to its own benefits, or at worst, grows up with the same issues as every other clothed child.